Excessive Crying in Infancy

For Margaret, Jennifer and Ciaran

Excessive Crying in Infancy

Tony Long

SRN, RSCN, RNT, BSc (Hons), MA, PhD

Senior Lecturer in Child Health
Centre for Nursing, Midwifery and Collaborative Research
University of Salford

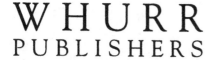

WHURR
PUBLISHERS

© 2004 Whurr Publishers Ltd
First published 2004
by Whurr Publishers Ltd
19b Compton Terrace
London N1 2UN England and
325 Chestnut Street, Philadelphia PA 19106 USA

British Library Cataloguing in Publication Data
A catalogue record for this book is available from the
British Library.

ISBN 1 86156 449 X

Contents

Preface

> Roisin let the health visitor in and sat down. Scott contin-
> ued to scream in her arms. 'How is he?' asked the health
> visitor. 'I hate him!' shouted Roisin, bursting into tears.
> 'Take him away!'

For three years during the 1980s I worked as a charge nurse on a children's ward in a district general hospital. It was then that my interest
was first aroused in the issue of excessive infantile crying. Parents with
whom I had clinical contact told harrowing stories of their experiences,
and their distress and exhaustion were evident. A baby who cried
excessively seemed to exert profound effects on the family's quality of
life and appeared adversely to affect the health of all those living in the
household.

As this interest matured later in my professional life I began to take
more notice of promotional literature for colic remedies and other
sources of information for parents. I became increasingly concerned
about the common over-simplification of complex physiological and
clinical issues; the enthusiasm of claims for a panacea; and the careless
recommendations for parents to pursue radical interventions without
evidence of medical necessity and without the benefit of professional
advice. While there was, and still is, a huge amount of literature on the
cause and cure of excessive infantile crying, work relating to the way
that parents cope with the crying seemed remarkably lacking. Clearly,
cure in such cases would normally be far better than having to cope, but
in many cases a cure is simply not to be found, and parents have to find
a way to get through the experience until the crying eventually abates.
It was such cases that prompted my own research into excessive infantile crying and which form the subject of this book. Specifically, it is
about parents coping with excessive crying (whether or not from colic
– whatever that might be) in children of less than one year of age.

Despite significant advances in medical knowledge, excessive crying continues to be a common problem which exerts serious effects on many families, adversely affecting their quality of life and causing great distress. Myth and misunderstanding surround the problem, exacerbating the difficulties and hampering better-informed efforts to help. In an age of widespread access to the Internet and a multitude of media messages it is all too easy to be persuaded by assertions that are at best misguided, often simply wrong, and at worst actually harmful.

Searching for 'infant crying' or 'crying baby' on the world-wide web using any commonly used search engine will quickly reveal numerous sources of detailed advice and self-declared expert knowledge. 'Dissolve a hard peppermint candy in a warm bottle of water'[1] advises one Internet site. Presumably one of the ingredients is thought to be helpful, but when I tried it the water was cold long before the 'hard candy' had dissolved, and looking at the ingredients of most such sweets, they are not inviting as medicine for a baby.

Examples like this are more likely to be a waste of time than harmful, but other examples may cause completely unnecessary and intense distress. Referring to the mother who declines to attend immediately to a baby crying for no apparent reason, another expert says, 'Very early maternal neglect, in particular, has been shown to produce an undersized orbitofrontal cortex ... the baby grows up literally unable to feel guilty about hurting others.'[2] Such a scandalous assertion is not only factually wrong in this context, but is certainly not designed to support exhausted, anxious parents who are already likely to feel guilty and inadequate about their inability to pacify their infant.

If help is to be offered to parents then this needs to be based on sound understanding of the problem including physiological processes, the latest evidence on potential causes and treatments, and the perspective offered by the parents of what is problematic about the crying and what they want the help to address.

Before embarking upon the daunting task of improving the lives of families coping with a crying baby the health professional needs to be aware of the existing evidence – its content, its relative strength and its limitations. There is now a great deal of literature, and within this a significant and growing amount of research evidence. Some of this, as is often the case, is inexplicably poor, but other research studies can be seen to offer evidence which is convincing to varying degrees. Being familiar with the available evidence will clearly lend confidence to the health professional in judging how to intervene, and it will also serve as a means to counter the copious nonsense which is liberally sprinkled throughout many lay sources of advice.

This book is based partly on one specific study about supporting parents in coping with excessive crying, but it takes into account other research evidence. The research literature is woven into the text. The book is aimed primarily at the health care practitioner seeking to offer support to parents, and it is meant to complement rather than to replace existing evidence-based medical interventions. As with many problems in life, those who have not experienced the trauma of life with a baby who cries incessantly probably will not ever really understand the phenomenon. This book is intended to offer some insights into the complexities of excessive crying in infancy, to review the available evidence on which to base decisions, and to propose some essential messages that parents might find helpful in their efforts to cope.

Notes

1. http://babyparenting.miningco.com/blcolic.htm
2. http://babyparenting.miningco.com/library/weekly/aa040100c.htm

Chapter 1
Introduction

Purpose of the study

My aim in the study was to understand something of the experience of living and coping with a baby who cries excessively. Within this there were several specific aspects that I wished to address. The first of these was to elicit from families what factors or circumstances caused the crying to be perceived as challenging or problematic. I wanted to know what professional help was available to them and how they had responded to this. Finally, I sought to discover what made coping more difficult and what interventions or factors tended to effect an improvement in coping ability. I did not seek to identify the cause of excessive crying, neither did I hold any hope of discovering a cure.

The sample

The participating families were recruited from families in West Yorkshire reporting excessive crying in their infant. The recruitment area included a large metropolis and a wide variety of urban, city-centre and rural areas. Inclusion criteria for recruitment to the study were restricted to three items. First, the baby currently crying had to be under one year of age. Beyond this age excessive crying is normally considered to be a behavioural problem since children should have the ability to make their feelings and desires known in a more constructive manner. Second, the identified problem had to relate to the baby reportedly crying excessively as perceived by the family. It did not matter whether or not the baby had been treated by any health care professional, or referred to one, and neither did the diagnosis of physical illness exclude the baby. This was because the perception of the problem and the means of coping were the important factors. Third, those to be interviewed had to speak English or have someone in the

home available to translate. The complexity of the issues under examination required clear communication. Apart from these restrictions,
anyone involved in caring for the baby or living in the household
whether parents, family, friends or paid help could be considered as
informants.

The final sample was made up of 14 families from which a total of 25
individuals were interviewed. On six occasions a single family member
(the mother on each occasion) was present, while another interview
was conducted with four family members. In addition to the 13 babies
who were currently crying excessively, another baby and a further six
siblings were discussed who had cried previously. One family was currently coping with its third crying baby. A total of nine siblings were
present, usually as a single addition, during eight of the interviews.

Some participants lived in run-down council housing estates, others
were from rural settings, and yet others from recently built, landscaped
estates containing four and five-bedroomed detached houses. This variety was evident within the selection of families from a major metropolis
as well as those from other towns, cities and rural locations elsewhere
in the county. The literature did not support any suggestion that the
factors which underpin the Registrar General's social classification were
of particular relevance (although Crowcroft and Strachan, 1997 found
some social factors to be associated with higher rates of mothers reporting colic). It was no surprise that families from minority ethnic groups
did not feature within the sample. There is evidence in the literature
that failure to recruit from such groups is common even to large, fund-
ed projects with access to hundreds or thousands of potential recruits
(St James-Roberts et al 1996, Barr et al 1988, Van der Wal et al 1998).
Within the geographical area considered for the study there were large
Asian communities. However, despite efforts to recruit from towns and
cities with recognised minority ethnic communities there were no
Asian, Chinese or African respondents, although a few Irish individuals and one other European parent participated.

Part of the sample was identified by health visitors from their own case-
loads. Families were approached with a view to recruitment either by
telephone or during a routine visit. Written details of the study were provided and time allowed for reflection before deciding to participate. This
sampling approach would be labelled 'selective' by some, or 'nominated'
by others. The remaining informants were included after responding to
posters displayed in baby clinics, on general notice-boards in health
centres, an accident and emergency department, a GP surgery, and a paediatric out-patient clinic. This approach is often said to result in a
'volunteer' sample.

Data collection

Data collection was mainly through semi-structured interviews. However, data were also collected by means of a questionnaire, and there was a considerable amount of observational data included in field notes.

The questionnaire was designed primarily to save time at the interview by establishing factual details such as family make-up and housing style. Other items provided material which could be useful should the conversation flag during the interview. These related to listing the three most important effects on the family, or words that would be used to describe the family's reaction to the crying. The questionnaire was structured in three sections over four sides of A4 paper and comprised 40 questions. The three sections dealt with issues about the baby (20 questions); the rest of the family (10 questions); and professional help (10 questions). Most items were closed questions requiring only a tick in a box or entry of a number. A few (7) required the respondent to chose one or more boxes to tick, while others (10) required the respondent to compose the answer. In these questions the space provided indicated that no more than six words would be expected. Piloting of the questionnaire indicated that answering all but these 10 questions would commonly take less than five minutes. The remaining questions might require approximately 10 minutes to complete.

The interviews were conducted at informants' houses at a time convenient to them. One informant preferred to be interviewed at work and another opted to be interviewed at the university. Part of the encounter was tape-recorded using a Walkman-sized recorder. A single visit was made to each household and the time spent there varied from a minimum of 90 minutes to a little more than three hours on one occasion.

The time spent in taped interview ranged from 45 minutes to 90 minutes, with additional time spent in more informal discussion, observation, and participating briefly in the family's life after the tape recorder was switched off. The opportunity to engage in participant observation arose partly from participants' desire to offer a more accurate and thorough picture of life with the problem and probably also from the availability of someone who had time and wanted to understand more. Participation in this case involved helping with child care and domestic tasks (like washing up), sharing a snack, chatting about family life, and other mundane aspects of life at home with a baby. On occasion it also included offering advice or information about propri-etary medicinal products or infant nutrition.

Field notes were not normally recorded during the taped interview time, although items were scribbled down discreetly at other times during the period of participant observation. In addition, hasty notes were always made shortly after leaving the house before memory faded or imagination could remodel recollection. More thoughts were noted as potential connections and avenues of investigation came to mind. Notes taken in close proximity to the interviews and those made later between episodes of formal data collection were eventually treated uniformly as data. Use was made of the memo facility in QSR NUD*IST. Data collection occurred over a period of slightly less than 12 months.

Data analysis

Data analysis followed an iterative process making use of the grounded theory techniques of open coding, constant comparison and theoretical sampling, and utilising the software package QSR NUD*IST 4. Preliminary analysis was undertaken of each interview as it was concluded and transcribed, together with the corresponding questionnaire answers and any field notes, amending the emerging understanding of the issues, and used to inform subsequent interviews. Axial coding was pursued in a novel manner through the use of concept maps, continually adjusting and amending these as the interviews progressed and the emerging theory developed. This was continued into an analytical phase with the same purpose as selective coding in grounded theory which resulted in the final theoretical conclusions.

Ethical issues

Consent was gained in a formal, written manner, emphasising the voluntary nature of participation and the absolute right to withdraw from the study at any time. Printed details were posted to the informants together with the questionnaire. There was no element of deception involved in the study and approval was secured from a major local research ethics committee. Confidentiality was assured by the anonymising of the transcripts and questionnaire responses. Contact details of the participants were recorded manually on paper and stored separate from the data and other study materials. Informants were not referred to by name or number in subsequent reports. Each informant was also given the choice to have the tape recording erased on completion of data analysis.

Chapter 2
The nature and size of the problem

Excessive crying or colic?

Although there are earlier references in the literature, certainly as early as 1921 according to Illingworth (1954), it is generally accepted that two concurrent papers in 1954 represented the first formal recognition of excessive crying as an entity worthy of medical investigation. These seminal works, which are easy to criticise today (50 years later) on grounds of lack of rigour, were suitably academic in their day, and they were important contributions in stimulating interest, debate and research into this topic.

Illingworth (1954) presented details of his study which introduced the term 'three months colic', defining this as 'a clinical entity in which the baby, in the first three months of life, has rhythmical screaming attacks in the evenings, which are not stopped when he is picked up, and for which there is no obvious explanation, such as hunger'. He added that he considered severe episodes 'to be so characteristic that they cannot be confused with anything else'. A wide range of suggested causes were dismissed (including feeding problems, mismanagement, allergy, swallowed air, and foods taken by the mother), and 'local obstruction to the passage of gas in the colon by local spasm or kinking of uncertain cause' was thought to be the probable explanation. In fairness, Illingworth later revoked this proposition, noting that although gastro-intestinal pathology is commonly held to be responsible for colic, no evidence had then been provided for this (Illingworth 1985). The idea of a three months deadline is now firmly fixed into lay beliefs about infant crying. The notion of colic as an unambiguous clinical diagnosis is now less widely accepted, while all of the potential causes dismissed by Illingworth have been proposed again in more recent studies.

By a remarkable coincidence, an alternative perspective on the same clinical phenomenon was published in the same year in an American journal. Wessel et al (1954) preferred the term 'paroxysmal fussing'.

Table 2.1: Grading of fussiness (from Wessel et al 1954).

Contented	No paroxysms of crying (or at least fewer than below)
Fussy	Otherwise healthy and well-fed, has paroxysms of irritability, fussing or crying lasting for a total of more than three hours per day on more than three days in any one week.
Seriously fussy	'Fussy' paroxysms recurring for more than three weeks, or so severe that medication was indicated.

The researchers graded the degree of 'fussiness' as in Table 2.1.

The authors noted that 'seriously fussy infants would be classified as "colicky" by most pediatric observers'. Despite the admitted arbitrary fixing of a threshold for serious fussing, the 'rule of threes', as the criteria became known, continues to be the most commonly accepted definition of colic in clinical practice and in research. However, many alternative criteria are used (particularly in research), and this has led to difficulty in interpreting and comparing results from various studies. For example, the criteria were modified by Carey (1992) to require the crying to persist for four days per week (a criterion used by others, too). Suggestions of intestinal pathology were avoided, however, and the term 'primary excessive crying' was preferred to colic. Carey also adopted Illingworth's criterion of the baby being otherwise healthy and well-nourished, and the additional distinction was introduced that the crying should be 'at full force'. No further explanation of what constitutes 'full force' was provided.

The effects of using varying definitions on sample size and nature as well as on results was shown particularly effectively in a large study in The Netherlands by Reijneveld et al (2001). The parents of 3,345 infants of less than six months were interviewed to establish the length of time for which the infant cried over recent periods. The cases were then assigned to one or more categories according to the fit with 10 published definitions of excessive crying. The outcome was that the same population would yield widely differing samples in response to the application of the 10 definitions. Study findings, therefore, are strongly influenced by the selected definition of excessive crying. The mixture of arbitrary criteria of duration of crying and vague notions of intensity characterises many attempts to define and investigate excessive crying and colic.

St James-Roberts (1991) has suggested that there are three apparent applications of the term 'colic'. The first relates to the infant's behaviour: the amount and intensity of crying, and this corresponds with a preference in terminology of 'persistent crying'. The difficulty with this mode of definition is that there is no meaningful threshold for the transition from elevated but still normal levels of crying to abnormal, excessive levels. This problem was expressed clearly by Barr et al (1992) and supported by data from eight studies.

> Delineation of a colic syndrome is made more difficult by similarities between the crying behaviour of infants with and without colic. In particular, daily duration of crying in normal infants tends to increase until the second month of life and cluster during the evening hours, a pattern typically reported for infants with colic. This has understandably raised the question as to how much crying is 'normal' and whether the crying of colic is distinctly different or simply the upper end of a spectrum of otherwise normal crying.

So colic may refer not to a clinically distinct group of crying infants but simply to those in the upper echelon of normal crying.

For one study Barr and his colleagues defined colic instead as 'a clinical complaint' (Barr et al 1992). This meant that crying which was considered problematic by mothers was labelled as colic. The study then investigated the correlation between various groups of infants on a large number of social and physiological characteristics. On these terms, significant differences were found between infants which satisfied the requirements for Wessel's colic and those which did not. The sole difference with regard to crying, however, was that the colicky infants sustained longer bouts of crying. There was nothing to support any suggestion of differences in total amount of time spent crying or in the sound of the cry. This approach to defining colic represents St James-Roberts' (1991) second option. What both he and Barr et al accept is that this approach is reliant upon maternal attributes and is highly unstable and variable across cases. Once again, the central phenomenon of the amount of crying does not distinguish between 'excessive or persistent crying' and 'colic'.

St James-Roberts' final suggested use of the term 'colic' differs from the previous two in that where they were largely descriptive the third is more explanatory in nature. The root of the word colic is in its Greek adjectival form *kolikos* referring to intestinal involvement. Pain resulting from gastro-intestinal malady is often held to be the defining cause of colic. There is, however, little consensus with regard to the specific intestinal problem underlying colic. Moreover, in a later study (St James-Roberts et al 1996) it was found that most infants who met Wessel's colic criteria showed no signs other than excessive crying. This large study, which was well-designed and compared babies rated as persistent criers, evening criers and moderate criers on defined characteristics labelled 'fussing', 'crying' and 'having colic', was limited to a degree by half of the sample failing to complete diaries as required and an under-representation of mothers from Asian or Afro-Caribbean origin. Both of these issues represent persistent problems in such research however well-planned and conducted. Nevertheless, a remarkable under-reporting of colic was found in this study. Of those infants who were gauged to meet Wessel's rule of three only 35% were reported as having colic by the mother. The results appear to provide clear evidence that, with regard to signs of colic, the correlation between infant behaviour and maternal perception is often hopelessly unreliable. Furthermore, the defining feature of colic being paroxysmal was dismissed entirely both by data from diaries and from audio recordings. Such bouts of colic as could be recognised did not commence paroxysmally and could not be distinguished from other episodes of crying by their preceding characteristics. This tends to support the notion that colic is not a separate clinical entity or a distinguishable sub-group of crying behaviour.

The net result of these deliberations is that 'excessive crying' or 'persistent crying' are preferable to 'colic' as descriptors of the crying behaviour under consideration. 'Colic' bears notions of intestinal pathology, which often cannot be verified, is ambiguously defined, and is extremely difficult to differentiate from excessive crying as a clinical entity. However, much of the available evidence about excessive crying has been undertaken using 'colic' as a descriptor (often, clearly, erroneously), and it would be foolish to ignore such sources of knowledge. With so little agreement on the definition of the problem, and with the difficulties endemic to definitions flawed by artificial thresholds and ambiguous terminology, it is hardly surprising that great difficulty is encountered in establishing the rate of excessive crying or colic.

Patterns of excessive crying

Surprisingly, in view of the data available for other aspects of an infant's anatomy, physiology and behaviour, before the study by St James Roberts and Halil (1991) there was no reliable standard for 'normal' crying. The results from this study, parts of which confirmed an otherwise fragmented record in the literature, established what is now accepted as the baseline standard for infant crying. The findings are summarised in Table 2.2. Similar work has now been completed in relation to normal sleep patterns (Bartlet and Witoonchart 2003).

The difficulty with establishing an upper limit of normality to the amount of time spent crying remains. The details above go a long way towards clarifying the pattern of normal crying. St James-Roberts and

Table 2.2: Baseline Standard of Normal Crying (From Golton and St James-Roberts 1991).

1 Crying is at its maximum in the first three months. An average of about two hours crying per day is to be expected. This average halves between four and 12 months.

2 Crying peaks at about six weeks (although with considerable individual variation).

3 In the first three months the crying clusters in the late afternoon and evening. The hours between 6pm and midnight account for 40% of the 24-hour total.

4 From about six months the afternoon/evening clustering disappears and the pattern changes to one of an increase in night-time crying for the last quarter of the first year. The night-time peak is less common than the afternoon/ evening peak and occurs mostly in those babies who cry for longer periods anyway.

5 Most babies cry for 30 minutes or less in any period of the day. (These periods are defined as morning, afternoon, evening and night.)

Halil (1991) were able to demonstrate that babies who were referred by their parents to the GP or health visitor followed the same pattern of crying as 'normal' babies. The major differentiating factor (verified by the use of audio-recording) was that parents reported the amount of crying to be two or three times greater than the average. Crying usually occurred during every period of the day (but with a peak in the afternoon and evening). No birth order or sex differences were found to be relevant. This is important as lay knowledge commonly asserts that male children are more likely to cry excessively. Although excessive crying is no more common in first-born children, it is more common for first-time parents to seek professional assistance with the crying. These findings were strongly supported by McGlaughlin and Grayson (2001) in a study with 297 mothers designed specifically to test previous study results.

The next step was obviously to compare clinically referred cases with the normative data. Making use again of diaries and audiotapes, St James-Roberts et al (1993) compared the crying duration of 16 referred infants at six weeks and 16 'normal' infants in a control group with the norm established above. In the researchers' words:

> These findings provide the first objective, tape-recorded evidence that mothers who seek advice from professionals for infants' excessive crying are correct in believing that their babies cry substantially more than average.

Another study by Baildam et al (1995) also sought to establish normative data on crying patterns. Diaries were used for 24-hour periods with 174 mothers together with semi-structured interviews on the following day. Strategies were employed to enhance the quality of diary recording (such as a dry-run before discharge from hospital) and this appeared to be effective. The poor compliance experienced in previous studies was largely overcome, and the follow-up interviews were used to check on gaps in the data. As with St James-Roberts et al (1993), it was found that mothers who reported excessive crying did, indeed, have babies who cried significantly in excess of the normal expectation. The study also found the expected peak in crying at about six weeks with a gradual decline thereafter. Two aspects, however, differed from previous findings. There was no evidence of the crying pattern changing to one of night-time crying in the last quarter of the first year. The meaning of this in previous work is questionable, anyway. Of more significance was the absence of an evening peak in crying. The authors suggest two possible explanations for this. In contrast to most other studies, fussing was discounted so that only active crying was recorded. If the evening peak were to be accounted for by fussing rather than crying then the results from this study would be compatible with others. However, the study by St James-Roberts and Halil (1991), for example, included discrimination of intensities of crying and still found a clear evening peak. An alternative explanation for this result seems more plausible. Crying behaviour was addressed in the study only as part of a wider investigation of postnatal development and within the context of other activities. 'It is possible that if mothers are asked to keep diaries specifically to record infant crying, they may even anticipate an evening peak' (Baildam et al 1995). Why the mothers should selectively (even though presumably subconsciously) deviate from valid entries for the evening peak requires more explanation. One Australian study also differs on this issue from the majority. Hill et al (1992), using the standard combination of diaries and audiotape, also failed to find the evening peak of crying. However, as with Baildam et al, this could be accounted for by their restriction of data collection to a single 24-hour period for each infant which has been shown previously to lead to erroneous results (Barr et al 1988).

Several studies have considered patterns of crying in other countries. The correlation in the pattern and intensity of normal crying between the studies by Michelsson et al (1990) and St James-Roberts and Halil (1991) is striking. The correlation for crying in the first three months (including a peak at six weeks) is also supported by studies in Canada (Hunziker and Barr 1986) and (although now rather old data) in the USA by Brazelton (1962). The latter study, in particular, was less clear on the issue of what counted as crying. Fussing is often included with crying (and often used interchangeably) in studies, but Brazelton's study included babies whose only crying-type activity was fussing which he defined as 'whimpering in a discontented fashion'. This is most certainly different to 'crying in full force'. Despite this it is clear that the weight of evidence upholds the notion of a standard pattern of crying at least in western countries. Work with infants in Denmark (Alvarez and St James-Roberts 1996) and India (St James-Roberts et al 1994) also supports this. Additional evidence is supplied by Barr et al (1996) in a study using diaries over a number of days and including fussing with crying that premature infants comply with the same normal crying pattern. This is an important finding since it indicates that 'this pattern represents a behavioural phenomenon that is universal to the human species' (Barr et al 1996). This seems to be a little ambitious since the studies involved have all been directed at western societies. Indeed, there is evidence that infants in other (eastern) societies may display different patterns of crying behaviour (Lee 1994). Nevertheless, for European, North American and other 'western' countries the pattern holds true. Establishing patterns of normal crying and identifying instances which exceed this in intensity does not, however, address the issue of how common excessive crying might be. There have been as many attempts to gauge the rate of excessive crying as there have to define it.

Incidence of excessive crying

As with efforts to establish the normal pattern of infantile crying, European contributions to the debate are helpful. Michelsson et al (1990) examined 'normal' crying times before considering aberrant cases, concluding that 9% of mothers in Sweden required help with a crying baby. Importantly, they recognised the crucial nature of the parents' perception of whether or not the crying was problematic, and found that this perception was justified by the amount of crying actually recorded.

In Finland, Lehtonen and Korvenranta (1995) investigated the possibility of seasonal variation in the incidence of excessive crying but found no such variation. Adopting Wessel's definition of colic they used diaries for at least one week per infant with 959 families to record time spent in normal crying and in colicky crying. The control group of infants complied well with the normal crying pattern detailed above, while the colicky group differed only in the intensity of the crying. An overall incidence of colic was recorded at 13% in healthy, full-term infants. Since colic was defined only by Wessel's rule of three, there is no reason to prevent this figure being interpreted as the incidence of excessive crying.

A different picture emerged from a study in Sweden, however. Canivet et al (1996) undertook a study with 152 mothers in a diary recording group and 224 mothers interviewed retrospectively. Four definitions of colic were employed and used for analysis.

Colic A: Wessel's colic.
Colic B: Barr's amendment of this (Barr et al 1992), with the three weeks criterion or the criterion of medical intervention replaced by a criterion of one week.
Colic C: Actual crying/screaming for at least one hour/day on four days/week (as per Carey 1992).
Colic D: Parental perception of colic (as per Barr et al 1992).

This complex design, perhaps not surprisingly, led to complex results. True Wessel's colic was found to have an occurrence rate of 9.3%. However, the four definitions produced incidences ranging from 8.5% (Colic D) to 16% (Colic C). The remaining group (Colic B) had an incidence of 11.7%. The mean incidence was, then 11.4%. However, the researchers interpret the results to indicate that colic may be less common than other studies commonly suggest. Herein, of course, lies the greatest difficulty in addressing the incidence of excessive crying or colic. Varying definitions produce varying results. Canivet et al demonstrate this within a single study. Their suggestion that colic may have become less common than previously must, therefore, be treated with caution. All of the four definitions used in this study have been used at some point in the studies whose results Canivet et al use as comparisons. There were additional problems with the study which limit confidence in the validity of the findings. Importantly, response rates were particularly low. Of 409 potential recruits invited to participate in completing diaries, 200 were unwilling to comply. Of the remaining 209, 48 failed to complete the diary, six diaries were 'lost in the mail', and three were excluded for other reasons. This left only 152 out of the original 409: a major issue when considering the representative nature of the sample. In fairness, the researchers admit this and attempted to combat the problem by introducing retrospective interviews with all those from the 409 who failed to complete a diary. This proved more successful in that 224 out of a possible 254 were recruited. However, the interviews were conducted when the infant was five to seven months old. Since the data required related to the amount of crying during the first three months this provided ample scope for faulty recollection and other hazards to accuracy. Although the study provides a great deal of food for thought, the results must remain suspect.

Van der Wal et al (1998) noted a rate of excessive crying in western countries of between 3% and 30%, but accepted that such an estimation was unavailable specifically for The Netherlands. A large study of 1,826 families in Amsterdam using retrospective questionnaires deliberately targeted a multi-cultural population with Dutch, Surinamese, Turkish, Moroccan and other families included. This factor affected response rates, clearly influenced the results, and gave rise to the greatest concerns about dangerous soothing practices (which will be addressed later in this book). In all, 7.6% of babies were reported to cry for three or more hours per day. Crying was reported to be a problem, however, by 20.3% of mothers. The researchers (justifiably) concluded that:

> Some parents cannot tolerate the least amount of crying, while others do not experience long crying periods as troublesome. Therefore, intervention efforts should be guided by parents' perceptions of infant crying, irrespective of the actual amount. (Van der Wal et al 1998)

Estimates continue to appear (eg Søndergaard et al 2000), but little of a convincing nature can be drawn from the plethora of work available with regard to the incidence of excessive crying. The multitude of estimates is clearly as much a result of divergent definitions, varying samples, and differing methodological approaches as any clinical or epidemiological factor. Diaries kept by mothers are a favoured method of data collection, but the studies considered here have shown the difficulties associated with non-compliance and partial completion. Work by Barr et al (1988) has demonstrated that using diaries is a major commitment for the mother and that diaries are unlikely to be completed as required by substantial proportions of the population. This applies particularly to those of lower socio-economic status and those with poor educational achievement. A significant degree of skewing can be effected through selective compliance in recording diary data. Additional use of audiotaped data enhances confidence in such data. However, the method is onerous on parents at a time when they are already under increased stress. It is feasible that mothers with the most demanding circumstances and the greatest degree of difficulty in coping may have babies who cry the most but would be unable to find time to complete a diary (Golton and St James-Roberts 1991). Adjusted arrangements for time sampling and easier recording processes can enhance diary completion and compliance.

Retrospective interviews (when directed at quantitative measures) may increase the response rate but risk errors of recollection if undertaken more than a brief period after the event. Finally, questionnaire methods are notorious for poor response rates generally, and have not been widely used in this area. A final approach to establishing the dimensions of the problem of excessive crying diverges from any standard epidemiological method and considers instead how much time and effort is expended in responding to requests for help from parents who declare a problem with their baby's crying (Barr et al 1992, St James-Roberts 1993a, Van der Wal et al 1998). Messy though this might be, it seems to be the only realistic measure if responses to the problem are to be considered. While measures such as Wessel's criteria may be needed for much of the research into excessive crying, for clinical purposes crying is a problem if parents declare it to be so. Such parents, whatever the intensity of the crying, require professional intervention. The nature of this intervention, however, must be dependent partly upon the perceived explanation for the crying, and it is to this that the discussion proceeds.

Chapter 3
The search for a cause

Evidence in the literature

There is a wealth of literature addressing explanations of excessive crying and these can be grouped into three main approaches:

- Physiological disturbance
- Infant temperament and maternal response
- Deficiencies in parenting practices

Parents, too, invariably have notions of what has caused the excessive crying in their baby and they may expend enormous amounts of time and energy in seeking a diagnosis and a cure. Some examples of these parental responses will be explored after a review of the research evidence for potential causes of excessive crying.

Physiological disturbance

The greatest proportion of the literature addresses physiological causes of colic or excessive crying. A smaller part of this considers the possibility of a transient autonomic nervous system anomaly which adversely affects the infant's ability to modulate its response to normal stimuli (Lester et al 1990, DeGangi et al 1991). As Barr et al (1999) have suggested, the problem may be that the baby is simply unable to regulate the crying which commences as a normal response to internal or external stimuli. Excess activity of both parasympathetic and sympathetic branches has been hypothesised. Excessive sympathetic nervous system activity, for example, certainly provokes gastric and intestinal effects which could result in the sort of discomfort apparent in reported colic and excessive crying, while vagal predominance has been suggested in the earlier consideration of colic as a problem of hypertonia. Fairly tentative findings have resulted from studies such as these, with a need for considerably more confirmation before this explanation can be accepted. For example, demonstration of a mechanism to explain the common reduction in symptoms from around three months would be a significant development. A problem common to most such studies is the difficulty of separating key variables in very young infants, especially if premature or if the mother suffered complications of pregnancy. Moreover, Kirjavainen et al (2001) have shown in a small but well-conducted study that no difference was to be found between infants with or without colic in the balance of the parasympathetic and sympathetic nervous systems. Despite these problems there is clearly some potential in this line of investigation.

The bulk of the literature, however, relates to some aspect of cow's milk intolerance or gut motility. Inexplicably, many studies in this field appear to be limited by poor method and inadequate sampling. Wolke's review of some of these provides a telling critique (Wolke 1993). Lothe et al (1982), for example, found that 'cow's milk seems to be a major cause of infantile colic in formula-fed infants'. However, while the authors claim to have used a double-blind method involving randomised use of hydrolysed protein or soy-based formula, it is clear from the description in the report that the mothers in the study would have known which milk was being used. Since they were also aware of the study design and aims, the findings are distinctly suspect. In a subsequent study, Jakobsson and Linberg (1983) attempted to improve on this design, implementing a true double-blind crossover design, but again experienced difficulty with the sample. Although cow's milk protein allergy was again found to be a significant clinical problem, Wolke (1993) suggests that problems remained with regard to the sample which may have been skewed by an inordinate number of subjects with a family history of allergy.

Other studies have fared no better. Stahlberg and Savilahti (1986) employed a sample of only 10 infants in a double-blind crossover study investigating the effects of breast milk and cow's milk formula with and without added lactase. It seems naïve to expect that mothers would not recognise the difference between breast milk and cow's milk formula when used for a week each, so the blind nature of the study is certainly questionable. Moreover, the sample was made up of weaned infants with a mean age of almost 12 weeks, a significant proportion of whom might be expected to be emerging from the symptoms of colic or excessive crying.

Attempting to determine a correlation between colic and cow's milk protein intolerance, Iacono et al (1991) adopted a rather odd set of criteria to assess 'severe colic' in a sample selected from the most severe cases attending a gastroenterology outpatient clinic. Although 240 infants had been diagnosed with colic, only 70 were used for the study: those with the worst symptoms. The authors conclude that cow's milk protein intolerance is a causative factor of colic in 'a considerable percentage' of infants with severe colic. The utility of this finding is questionable since the distinction between colic and severe colic was simply the calculation of crying for four hours per day rather than for three hours per day (as in the 170 infants excluded from the study). If intolerance to cow's milk were a significant causative factor in colic it ought to be present in most cases, not simply in a selected minority of the most serious examples. The method of the study was also dubious, with participating mothers easily able to recognise which milk was being used and thereby be influenced in recording the data in daily diaries. Additional studies by Jakobsson et al (2000) and Estep and Kulczycki (2000) suffered from a serious limitation in sampling. The first of these used 15 infants taken from the worst colic cases available, while of the six cases included in the second study (pursuing the effectiveness of amino acid formula as a treatment for colic), one case had missing data, another was processed in a different manner, and a third revealed contrary results.

Other more rigorous studies have made more measured claims to the significance of their findings (such as Forsyth 1989), but the net result is a complete lack of consensus over the role of intolerance to cow's milk or its constituent parts in the aetiology of excessive crying. Clyne and Kulczycki (1991) reported that bovine IgG was present in greater quantities in the breast milk of mothers of babies with colic, but they employed a non-representative sample (mothers from the La Leche League), and the significance of this finding is unclear (although the implication was that the babies absorbed the implicated protein). A very large survey by Crowcroft and Strachan (1997) revealed no evidence of any significant connection between reported colic and dietary factors.

Despite a plethora of studies into aspects of gastro-intestinal pathology no conclusive advance has been made to date. Although Lehtonen et al (1994b) found a high incidence of hypocontractile gall-bladder in infants with colic, it was unknown whether this was a cause, effect, or coincidental feature of colic. Heine et al (1995) dismissed the suggestion of gastro-oesophageal reflux being likely to cause irritability in the first 12 weeks, but Berkowitz et al (1997) saw a correlation between this clinical finding and some cases of colic. Lothe et al (1990) found evidence of intestinal mucosal pathology in infants with colic (although the significance of this is unknown), but Lehtonen et al (1994a) could establish no difference in intestinal microflora between infants with colic and those without. Even greater confusion reigns over the significance of lactose absorption. Miller et al (1990) are unable to state whether their finding of increased breath hydrogen (an indication of incomplete lactose absorption) indicates a cause or an effect of colic.

Studies by Moore et al (1988) and Hyams et al (1989) established no difference in lactose absorption between infants with and without colic. Two small-scale but rigorously implemented double-blind studies have demonstrated the likelihood of transient lactose intolerance as a cause of excessive crying in some infants. Kearney et al (1998) and Kanabar et al (2001) employed pre-incubation of feeds with lactase to show reduction in crying in a proportion of infants with symptoms of colic. Importantly, measured claims are made by these two studies that in some cases crying can be reduced (rather than cured).

Reviewing the whole range of studies into potential gastro-intestinal features of colic, Miller and Barr (1991a) concluded that 'Gut pathology may, at best, explain a minority of cases. Although evidence ... exists, it is frequently undermined by methodologic limitations, notably inadequate definition of the subjects studied.'

Maturation or developmental issues form the basis of the remaining potential physiological explanations for excessive crying. The argument has been put most clearly by St James-Roberts (1993b) who suggests that fundamental developmental reorganisation taking place at key points in the infant's life may be responsible for excessive crying. This theory has also been supported by Barr (1990). In this hypothesis difficulty during the transition from one neurobehavioural developmental state to another is held to be expressed by excessive crying. Some have considered the genesis of mother–infant interaction to be the crucial factor, while issues relating to the development of the autonomic nervous system have also been held accountable (Lester et al 1990). St James-Roberts (1993b) has suggested the possibility of the transition from a four-hourly sleep–wake cycle to a diurnal rhythm stimulating the excessive crying. Each of these explanations is commensurate with features such as a major alteration in the crying at about three months (when significant developmental changes are known to be active). Problems remain, however, with such explanations. While links may be apparent, the evidence for developmental changes causing excessive crying is yet to be found. Similarly, it is not clear why only selected infants should be affected. Furthermore, developmental problems normally appear as delays rather than traumatic events, and the effects tend to be longer-lasting rather than resolving in just a few weeks. Nevertheless, this approach holds some promise for further research.

Infant temperament and maternal response

Suggestions of individual predisposition to certain behaviours or responses, common enough in the literature, were introduced formally by Thomas and Chess (1968, 1977) and the influential New York Longitudinal Study (NYLS) which was commenced in 1956. Although troublesome crying was considered within the study, a much broader framework of behaviours formed the basis of the definition of 'difficult temperament'. Nine wide-ranging dimensions of temperament were identified. Unfortunately, this work has repeatedly been misinterpreted and applied to problematic infant crying; work by Jacobson and Melvin (1995) being one example. This study exhibited several other problems, particularly defining colic as 'crying that occurs in the first four months of life' and addressing the study to infants between four and eight months old. Wessel's criteria for colic were said to be used, but the criteria were misinterpreted – a common phenomenon in research into infant crying; a small convenience sample of 55 babies (25 in the colic group and 30 in the non-colic group) was used; and a response rate of 33% to a questionnaire further weakened the findings. A more rigorous study by Barr et al (1989) to establish whether feeding choice and infant temperament were predictors of excessive crying produced equivocal results, and the researchers could conclude only that 'early infant temperament predisposes to early crying and fussing but is of limited use as a clinical predictor'. Temperament could be linked to the daily duration of crying (an important aspect of defining excessive crying) but not to the frequency of the crying, and there was no association between temperament and an evening peak of crying. Although crying babies may demonstrate irritable temperaments, great care must be taken not to assume causal relationships without further evidence. As St James-Roberts (1993b) has argued, 'the NYLS provides no direct evidence that difficult temperament underlies persistent crying'. The authors of the NYLS themselves indicate that additional elements of difficult temperament which might be expected to be present in excessive crying are notably absent (Thomas et al 1982). Just as with developmental problems, underlying temperamental factors would be expected to persist whereas excessive crying tends to abate within six months or so and certainly within the first year. In fact, Canivet et al (2000) thought they had found such a result, but of seven attributes examined at four years only one (temperament) was found to be any different for the ex-colic group, and this had been measured using an amended version of an established instrument, so the findings were not entirely convincing.

Medoff-Cooper (1995) noted that 'infants who experience colic generally are not difficult to manage during their non-crying hours' and concluded that 'colic should not be equated with a difficult temperament'. Sometimes the complexity of the relationship between infant temperament and infant–mother attachment causes circular arguments in the literature. Medoff-Cooper (1995) demonstrated this in a competent review of the literature on infant temperament in the first year.

Fish et al (1991) found that excessively crying infants whose mothers rated them as 'irritable' received less sensitive interaction from their mothers, thus suggesting that excessive crying causes a poor relationship and adversely affects maternal attachment. However, findings from Mangelsdorf et al (1990) suggested that maternal characteristics are the decisive factor in establishing a positive relationship, and infant temperament plays only a minor role in this.

There are more radical offerings within this group of theories. Laying claim to insight into the psyche of the baby, several writers identify the cause of excessive crying as interpersonal psychological conflict within the infant although the evidence for this is entirely lacking. Some make more outrageously extravagant claims. Jayachandra (1988) asserted that young infants feel frustration, resentment and distrust of parents who fail to follow his recommendations for care (expressed as five basic principles). The resultant mental stress, claimed Jayachandra, has the immediate effect of excessive crying, later manifested as asthma, violence and social unrest. No empirical evidence whatsoever was offered for these assumptions and accepted theory on each of these issues negates Jayachandra's assertions. Such irresponsible assertion does nothing to further understanding of excessive crying.

Deficiencies in parenting practices

Inadequate or unresponsive parental care has commonly been held responsible for excessive infantile crying. As with efforts to isolate infant temperament as a causative factor, the evidence is somewhat confusing and contradictory. Whether or not mothers of babies with colic or excessive crying are more anxious or lacking in parenting skills has been argued for many years. Paradise (1966) and Carey (1968) are surprisingly often quoted in the debate (see Pinyerd 1992, for example), although these studies are now over 30 years old. More recent evidence from Taubman (1988) demonstrated that counselling of mothers was more effective than changing the baby's milk in reducing the amount of crying. The implication drawn from this was that colic is the result of maternal misinterpretation of the baby's crying. However, it was possible that mothers simply coped better as a result of additional support rather than the crying itself abating. Pinyerd (1992), too, found that mothers of babies with colic were more generally anxious and stressed than those with 'normal' babies. She then proposed that 'such a response would result in a mother who is less emotionally available for her infant'. However, as Pinyerd admitted, there is a pressing need to distinguish between variables which are attributable to the mother and those which reside within the baby. It is possible that the crying provokes maternal anxiety and distress rather than the reverse. Evidence from longitudinal studies which might indicate whether or not mothers were anxious before the crying began (or perhaps before birth) remains lacking. Miller and Barr (1991b) have offered some evidence that maternal depression before or after birth has no effect on either the amount of crying or on care practices. Furthermore, Hubbard and Van IJzendoorn (1991) investigating in a rigorous study the effect of delayed maternal response on infant crying found no correlation with the duration of crying although there may have been a correlation with the frequency of crying. A particularly important finding was that parents often make a rational decision to delay responding to their infant following judgement of other signals and interpretation of the crying. A delayed response was not necessarily an indication of poor parenting. In practice it is not the speed of response that matters but the quality or appropriateness of the response. Keefe et al (1996), too, found that reduced interaction in the case of mothers of babies with colic might be an adaptive response in avoiding over-stimulation.

Evaluation of interventions based on parental behaviour modification has proved disappointing. Hunziker and Barr (1986) considered the effectiveness of supplementary carrying in reducing crying only to find that little effect was to be seen once the baby was already crying excessively. A study by Barr and Elias (1988) of inter-feed interval and maternal responsivity was no more successful. Although feeding more frequently and attending more quickly produced the result of quieter infants with less fretting and crying, this held true only with a sample whose parenting behaviour differed considerably from the societal norm.

Perhaps the most obvious problem with inadequate care as an explanation of excessive crying is that previously experienced parents may encounter problems with subsequent infants. Birth order has been shown to make no difference to the likelihood of excessive crying (St James-Roberts and Halil 1991). Furthermore, there is some evidence that parents of crying babies make more effort than usual to soothe their babies (St James-Roberts 1989, 1993b). Overall, the weight of evidence is that inadequate parental care is unlikely to cause excessive crying, and excessive crying is more likely to provoke greater efforts on the part of parents to deal with the problem.

The search for a diagnosis

While there was disagreement among the informants on some issues, all were agreed on one effect of the crying: they could not give up the search for a diagnosis.

3.1: Francis – There had to be something else

Maybe if someone had told me that there wasn't an answer I could have accepted it. I felt sure I'd done everything there was to do, and tried everything there was to try, but I couldn't help feeling like there had to be something else. I had to carry on looking for the answer.

It is, of course, highly questionable whether being told that there was no diagnosis for the crying would really have been accepted. The reluctance to give up hope and the irresistible determination to continue searching for the cause of the crying was often so intense as to be dysfunctional. Although parents recognised the futility of their efforts they felt unable to accept this reality.

It rules my life! It takes over my life. Doctors; paediatricians; lactulose; gripe water. It rules my life.

There have been times when my whole life has revolved around seeking explanations for the crying. From time to time, even recently, I've picked up the challenge to find out exactly what was causing it, but I've never managed.

Even in the face of persistent denial by doctors of any physical pathology in the baby, perhaps partly because of this, there was often a deep-seated reluctance to accept this state of affairs. The thought remained that the baby must cry for a reason, even if that reason could not be identified. The conflict between the necessity for a reason for the crying and the ability to identify and successfully remedy this reason was the crucial issue.

Some expressed their feelings with a fairly neutral attitude towards doctors, but others were more scathing. Such feelings of being fobbed off are addressed in detail in a later chapter, but for now it is sufficient to note the common lack of acceptance of negative findings by medical examination, and the constant search for a diagnosis to account for the crying.

Postulated reasons for the crying

A variety of suggested reasons for the crying were proposed by parents, sometimes in the form of weak hypotheses ('Sometimes I think she's bored'), and other times as reports of what had been considered and rejected. A sample of these is reproduced here to give a flavour of the total complement.

General discomfort

Not surprisingly, mundane aspects of child care were often implicated. Two features were particularly commonly considered: needing to keep the baby warm and the baby wanting to be held. After listing all that she had tried without success to date Susan explained her next plan.

> 3.2: Malachy – The need for warmth
>
> Well, the next thing to try in the pram will be a hot-water bottle. Or a heated electric blanket. If it's the warmth factor. They're the only two things left. He's had a fleecy blanket. He's laid on sheepskins. Sheepskin blanket and fleecy blanket. So that's next.

This gives some indication of the intensity and determination associated with attempts to find the cause. Every possible variation in the selected factor was pursued. In Susan's case, these were the last two elements in her current theory. If her efforts ran true to form, and once these interventions had failed, she would accept that the theory was false and settle back to a relatively stable state of acceptance until another theory presented itself.

Some parents pursued a different possibility. Rather than a need for warmth causing the crying perhaps it was simply a need to be held. For Joanne and her mother, Vivienne, it seemed that Mark simply needed to be held by anyone (and this was the only way to stop the crying, even temporarily), but they postulated an early root cause to this particular need.

> 3.3: Mark – The need to be held
>
> It could be a pair of robot arms as long as someone's holding him. After being in the special care baby unit because of prematurity he had a problem with keeping his temperature up, and then he had jaundice, so I never touched him for the first two weeks in hospital, and when he came home we only picked him up to feed him. And then we put him straight back down because we wanted him to conserve as much energy as possible. So for about four or five weeks he was never really held, and I put it down now, looking back, to that. Because he wasn't held, when

he is held now he's clinging to that, thinking, 'Oh, no. I
can't be put down.' And is that a sense of insecurity from
him being early?

Claire noted of Fleur in comparison to her son Jason (then 5) that

She just seems more gentle, somehow. She wants attention, too, but more just to have someone with her and
holding her than to be playing or tickling or whatever.

In this there was no suggestion of pathology, simply personal preference and individual difference between siblings.

Roisin's childminder, Cindy, too, found that carrying Scott around
was the only technique that achieved any temporary success in
quietening him, but she warned of a self-limiting aspect of this.

It's all right if you can spend hours and hours doing this
[indicating rocking and cuddling] but he's too heavy. It's
physically too much. And how do you get anything else
done like this, anyway? You'll end up hurting yourself.

A further element of holding and cuddling the baby to calm the crying was introduced by Stacy who habitually spent hours each day
holding Yvonne.

I think it's the closeness. Sloppy, aren't you [to Yvonne]?
But when she's not held she's rigid. If you put her down
she goes rigid and goes mad. When you pick her up again
it takes about 10 minutes before she calms down and settles again. She's sloppy. Soft.

Psychological causes and the baby's personality

Stacy hinted that there was more than a physical need to be held, and
that psychological or personality factors might play a part. There was a
discernible suggestion of this in other parents' stories, too. Some, however, were more forthright in suggesting psychological causes with
explicit declarations that the baby had no reason to cry: that the crying
was simply 'whingeing'.

3.4: Nicola and Mark – Whingeing and seeking attention

Even when she didn't have tummy-ache she still cried. She
was just a moitherer, weren't you? The screaming would

sometimes subside slowly or sometimes just stop like that [clicking fingers]. Now that wasn't for any cause. That was just whingeing.'   (Julie)

I know, I think, when the crying is just a whingeing cry and when there's something really wrong. To me, most of the time it's just whingeing. You know when you hear it … A half-hearted cry, like, can't be bothered too much. That's just whingeing.   (Joanne)

It was noticeable that men's response to the whingeing would be to leave the baby to carry on, perhaps staying with the baby and perhaps not.

If I think everything's all right with her, she's just whinge-ing. She may as well whinge in her cot than down here.'   (Mike)

Women deciding the baby was just whingeing would characteristical-ly continue to try to soothe the baby or to check again for an observable cause. This gender-related behaviour was identified and remarked on by six of the respondents, including both men and women. Not uncom-monly, an element of deliberate action was attributed to such needless crying. Sarah remarked of Patrick, '…There's other times when he cries and he just wants attention, and we're sussing that out a bit more now.' Andrew's father, Peter, struck a similar note, 'He's only five months but he knows if he starts playing up and crying, he knows that we'll pick him up for attention. There's nothing wrong: he just wants attention.'

Diane, Malachy's aunt, agreed that it was possible to know when the crying was solely to gain attention. 'You can tell the difference between a baby that's crying for pain, distressed, and a baby that's crying for attention. They start whining and whining and whining and crying and crying and crying. You can tell the difference in the pitch, can't you? And they can cry for half an hour for no reason at all. He does that. Already. He does that.'

3.5: Nicola – an unhappy personality

I thought she was going to be an unhappy child. I still do. She still whines a lot at you. And she's a cuddler. I think it's her personality. She loves cuddling. She lovely but she's not really a happy child.

Julie felt fairly resigned to the fact that Nicola was an unhappy child. Interestingly, when her three-year-old sister, Lucy, gave the researcher a piece of squashed banana Nicola immediately laughed, and throughout the period of participant observation she was seen to play and to smile. The notion of being an unhappy child was clearly meant to imply a general background personality rather than persistent behavioural discontent.

Deeper concerns about psychological causes (and effects) of the crying were revealed by others among the participants who had come to the decision that the crying might be simply a facet of the baby's personality. This was the case for Claire, who thought that Fleur's personality differed significantly from that of her five-year-old brother, and that it was her psychological make-up that caused her persistently to demand attention and close company.

Joanne expressed her belief that Mark might suffer in the long term because of an inability to enjoy life. 'Do you think that I might be right,' she asked, 'predicting that he will grow up to be less fun?' Despite the absence of any research evidence to support such a hypothesis she was not alone in her anxiety. Others voiced similar concerns.

Pain

Easily the most commonly suggested reason for the crying, proposed in some form by all but two of the respondents, was that the baby was in pain. This is not an isolated finding. St James-Roberts et al (1996) found that 75% of babies who cried excessively were thought to be in pain by their mothers. For the parents in this study the cause of the pain usually remained a mystery, but suggestions varied from teething to abdominal obstruction.

3.6: Patrick – he must surely be in pain

Well, the screaming seemed like he was in pain. It was – the only way I could describe it, really, was it just felt like the screaming was the fact that he was in pain. And the look on his face. Sometimes he wasn't even crying any more and he'd look at you as if to say, 'Do something!' But he really seemed to be in pain.

It was clearly an emotive issue, as was made explicit by Patrick's parents, Sarah and Richard. The research evidence for babies that cry excessively being in pain is, as yet, unconvincing, but acoustic analysis of such crying may demonstrate some characteristics compatible with crying resulting from painful procedures (Lester et al 1992). It was the thought that the baby might be in pain that caused the most guilt among parents, was the most difficult aspect of the crying to tolerate, and provoked the greatest dissatisfaction with the medical response.

Such expressions of guilt at not curing the crying were common, as were thoughts that the baby expected more from its parents. This aspect of interpreting the reason for the crying not just by the sound but also by additional behavioural features was considered by Fuller (1991). Rigorous testing demonstrated that acoustic differences between types of crying from pain, hunger and fussy crying were too small for humans to distinguish by sound alone. However, when the baby's facial expression and bodily movement were included, the possibility of discrimination increased substantially. Claire also thought that her baby, Fleur, cried with pain at least some of the time.

> Sometimes she would sound like she was in pain. Not most of the time, but sometimes. Yeah, it would sound like you'd just pricked her with a needle. She'd be happy and then suddenly she'd cry out and start. It's a bit like when they're teething and they get a sudden twinge out of the blue, and they start crying really hard, only she wasn't teething at all.

Phil and Eileen had been told that Rachel had colic but they were unconvinced.

> Eileen: Oh yeah. The only sign that we've been told was if they raise their knees it means they've got wind. But it's also a sign of pain, as well, isn't it? You know? I thought she was in pain, not just wind. I worried that I wasn't doing enough.
>
> Phil: There was no smile from her, you know. No. It was either she was asleep or she was in pain. Nothing else. And we thought, 'This can't be at all right.' She was in pain so much. It was just the worst time: the worst four months.

The emotional burden for parents was considerable, and it seemed to be made up of simple concern about the baby being in pain compounded by guilt at being unable to prevent or terminate the suffering. The concern and guilt could be relatively mild though persistent, as was the case for Stacy.

> It's like she's in pain, and no-one can comfort her. I know
> I've done everything that I can for her. We've tried every-
> thing. There's nothing more, but still she seems to be in
> pain. It wears me down a bit when it's day after day and
> night after night.

For others the episodes could be less frequent but far more disturbing. Helen recalled her struggle with Michael and her growing fears
that something was dreadfully wrong.

> Well, he must have been in pain. And when the pain
> stopped he got better. Sometimes it was just hard crying,
> what I would call hard crying. Other times it would be
> absolutely desperate: as though he was going to die. Like
> there was something terribly wrong with him... He'd be
> really red in the face and looking and sounding like he
> was going to expire.

So the fear that the crying was the result of pain was both intense
and widespread. Sometimes this concern was not much more than an
additional anxiety; for others it could be so intense as to represent
cause to fear for the baby's life. Five families readily remembered
having sought urgent medical intervention believing that their
baby's crying indicated serious organic pathology, possibly with the
baby's life at risk.

Feeding problems

Another common set of issues addressed both by professionals and parents related to problems associated with feeding and colic. More
specifically, the problems centred mostly around insatiable hunger; difficulties with breast-feeding; intolerance to breast or formula milk; and
expectations and understanding of colic. The possibility of each of
these being responsible for the crying was proposed on a fairly frequent
basis, and much time and effort was expended by parents on seeking
confirmation of the diagnosis or in establishing a cure. It was common,
too, for the focus to alter in the course of a few minutes from feeding
problems as a cause of the crying to feeding difficulties as a result of the
crying. This 'fog' of interchangeable issues relating to crying, feeding
and sleeping is a common phenomenon for health care professionals.
Every family included feeding problems and colic in some form in its
history of the crying.

3.7: Michael – Insatiable hunger

Food. That's all he was interested in. And then when he
wasn't feeding he was awake and crying. I was feeding him
myself. It was like an hour in every two feeding him for the
first few weeks. All day and all night. And that was the only
thing that would keep him quiet. You know, he'd go for 10
minutes after a feed and then he'd cry again. And I'd feed
him again. What else could I do? Nothing else worked.

So Helen found with Michael that the relief from the crying was
often short-lived. Despite evidence that the proposed solution was not
working, she persisted simply because there was no obvious alternative.

Claire, too, was particularly clear that Fleur must be hungry and
could be pacified only by being fed.

She was really inconsolable. The only way I could stop it
[the crying] was to feed her. I think partly, sometimes, it
was to do with hunger. We started her on solids at three
months rather than the suggested four months just to try
to stop the crying.

Such decisions to ignore professional advice were common although
not taken lightly. In some cases they may even be indicative of
advanced parenting skills, particularly since such strategies are resorted
to by health professionals, too.

Often the efforts to stop the crying would result in more and more
frequent feeding, perhaps with ever-greater amounts. This was usually
despite the parents' knowledge that the total amount of milk being
taken was well in excess of the expected requirement. Yet there had to
be a cause, and since the baby appeared to demand more milk, then perhaps more milk was needed. Joanne recounted this about feeding Mark.

3.8: Mark – Ever-increasing feeds

But then it just went to where he'd wake up in the morning and we'd give him his bottle. He'd have a nine ounce
bottle which was more than enough, and he'd carry on
crying. Nine ounces, yes. And he went on to 11 ounces,
because I kept on feeding him to stop him crying, to stop
him being so angry... I had to give up breast-feeding
because I couldn't keep up with the milk. He was just

demanding all the time. And all I was doing was expressing it and giving it to him in a bottle and then sterilising
bottles and so on. My day was just filled with it.

All three of the babies above, Fleur, Michael and Mark, were breast-
fed, and all had elder siblings who had also been breast-fed (indicating
that their parents were not novices). Indeed of the 14 babies in the
main study, seven were breast-fed. There are certainly popular myths
about the absence of excessive crying (and many other problems) in
babies fed on breast milk, but the experiences of the families in this
study suggest that breast-feeding is no protection against excessive crying. In contrast, breast-feeding could be an additional factor
contributing to the difficulties faced by parents. As before, the distinction between crying as cause or effect was at best vague.

Perhaps the epitome of determination to continue breast-feeding,
Elaine found the whole business of feeding Harry extremely trying and
unrewarding. She pondered the possibility of a lesion in the baby's
mouth causing pain on feeding.

3.9: Harry – A breast-feeding battle

…So he would start to feed and then he would stop and
cry and cry and cry and cry. We had him to the doctor's
and checked his mouth that there was nothing hurting
him when he was trying to feed. And all I could do was to
rock him to sleep and then, once he was asleep, try to
feed him again. I'd keep looking at the clock and thinking, 'Is he going to keep going, or is he going to start
crying again?' Usually, he would cry again. The whole
business was, like, stop-start, stop-start. So I'd be trying to
feed him, and rocking him to sleep, and trying again, and
so on. It could take ages to feed him. It seemed to be such
a struggle. It's particularly frustrating when you're feeding
him yourself. He ought to enjoy it, and I ought to enjoy it.
With James [then four years old] breast-feeding was
always a time when I sat down and relaxed and had a
drink. With Harry it's not like that. I still make a drink and
sit down, but… I try, but it's a battle.

Joanne and Eileen had different theories. For Joanne the problem
was not knowing how much milk Mark had taken and therefore being
unsure as to whether or not he was crying because he was still hungry.

I was feeding him one day and I thought, 'Right! I'm going
to see...' I was still breast-feeding then. And I was there an
hour and 20 minutes and he was still hungry, and I thought,
'I don't know how much he's had. So is he hungry? Or is
there something wrong with me?' Perhaps he was crying
because I wasn't producing milk properly for him or whatever. So I just thought, 'Oh, the bottle's so much easier and
at least I'll know what he's had.' Maybe it was my feeding
him that was causing the crying. It turned out that he cried
anyway, no matter what, so we'll never know.'

Producing sufficient milk was not a worry for Eileen. She had a more
sinister concern which caused her to cease breast-feeding and resort
instead to soya milk.

3.10: Rachel – The poisonous breast milk fallacy

Well, I used to try feeding her every time she cried. Because
she was bringing milk back up I thought she needed to
feed more. But I think there was also a bit of... Maybe I
needed to feel her feeding: doing something normal. And
maybe just me getting something right: doing something
she liked. I never minded the milk being wasted. So it was
partly for her but also partly for me to feel better. I think so,
anyway... But then I started to worry that I might be, like,
poisoning her with my own milk, so the good feeling about
doing something good for her went away.

Someone had suggested to Eileen that Rachel might be allergic to
her mother's milk and this had caused immense feelings of guilt. How
sad it was that such a natural and beneficial practice which both had
clearly enjoyed and which was evidently therapeutic to Eileen was no
longer available to them. Yet the nature of excessive crying seemed to
be that a cause must continually be sought, and even the most obviously innocent factor may become subject to suspicion and
prophylactic intervention.

Milk sensitivity

Changing the baby's milk because of suspected intolerance was a very
common strategy. Parents seemed happy to use the terms 'sensitivity',
'intolerance', and 'allergy' interchangeably although medically these
are discrete phenomena. The reason for changing milks and the

evidence of the need to do this remained vague. Julie's experience with selecting food for Nicola (her second child) was fairly typical. Each time she tried a new milk the crying continued or even became worse. It is noteworthy that the stimulus to change milks came from professionals, family and friends as well as from self-driven decisions and as a result of reading magazines. Julie also had an interesting view on keeping a final strategy in reserve (probably never to be used).

3.11: Nicola – Keeping something in reserve

She was on Farley's First, and then my friend told me to put her on Milupa, so I did. And then she said, 'Why don't you try her on the fuller, the hungrier one?' So I checked with the health visitor and she agreed and that's what I did. But it made her constipated. So that went out of the window. And then they [clinic] said to start her on weaner, which was at about 16 or 17 weeks. So I started her on weaner, but she got worse She was waking up in the night then, screaming her head off… A soya was one thing I didn't want to do because it was a last resort. If I put her on soya and it didn't work, I wouldn't have any lifelines left.

It was not only suspicion of sensitivity or intolerance to milk that provoked a change to soya formula. Susan changed Malachy's formula to Wysoy after hearing of her friend's experience with a baby suffering lactose intolerance. There was no indication of this being the case with Malachy, but the common lore of personal experience, culminating in the suggestion that 'it would be worth trying' is often a strong motivator, especially when there is no other solution on offer. However unlikely a suggested cause might be, it would be pursued in case this was the elusive factor that would indicate the diagnosis and consequent cure. Surprisingly, perhaps, finding that no improvement resulted from changing the milk often provoked not a search for an alternative explanation but, rather, a determination to try yet another brand or variety of milk formula or to proceed to early weaning. Janet and Peter actively sought a medical explanation. Their frustration with the medical response to the crying is indicative of the dissatisfaction often expressed by parents. This is dealt with in another chapter.

3.12: Andrew – Medical advice to change formula

Well Dr (GP) had put me on this Nutramigen [pre-digested formula] milk with Gaviscon in it. He'd settled on it. He

was still sick, but he was happier. And then I went to the
hospital a week after that and he took me off it because
that was the first time I'd gone to the hospital, and he said,
'Well, why is he on that milk?' I said, 'Well, my GP's put me
on it.' And he was going through a few reasons why and
everything. So he took me off that and put me on SMA
Gold and give me some other sort of medicine: a thicken-
er. And it was just... He totally went back to being a baby.
He was being sick all the time. Atrocious. So I went back
to my doctor the week after and I said, 'I can't stand this
any longer. He's crying all the time. He's worse now than
before. And the milk's done nothing.' And he just wanted
me to carry on for another week until I went back to the
hospital. So I went away and carried on with what the doctors at the hospital had told me, and I just waited until I
went there again, and then I told them how he had been.
And then he [hospital consultant] says to me, 'You should
have phoned me.' But he didn't say that to me before, so
I didn't know.'

Such perceived lack of agreement and consistent advice was not
uncommon. Roisin, too, had little joy in trying to establish a medical
cause for the crying. In addition to an episode in which, she reported,
a doctor had refused to speak to the family when they arrived at the
surgery with Scott screaming because he did not believe in milk intolerance, she summarised her other encounters.

3.13: Scott – Conflicting diagnoses and advice

They haven't agreed on what is wrong with him. We
have had five conflicting stories now. One doctor told us
it was just colic and that we just had to put up with it
and that he would grow out of it. And to make sure that
we had plenty of gripe water in the house. Another doctor has told us that he thought maybe it was milk
intolerance to the soya milk, and maybe he should go
onto the pre-digested. Another doctor told us that he
thought it was a blockage in the bowel that was causing
the problem. Another one then told us that it could be
a twisted bowel, and then, last night, the doctor at the
hospital told us that it was just constipation. Who do
you believe?

Seeking to establish a cause for the crying within the baby's diet would often result in ineffective intervention, multiple changes in milk type, early weaning, and, justified or not, frustration with medical practitioners. One aspect deserves special attention only because of its profile within the study and in the lives of the families involved. This is the diagnosis (if this is an appropriate term) of colic.

Colic

Colic has already been shown to be a clinically difficult term, surrounded by misunderstanding and confusion. Its use persists, however, and it is interesting to see what some parents understood by the term. Often, the diagnosis of colic would be made by the parents themselves without professional assistance. Joanne and her mother, Vivienne, did this.

> 3.14: Mark – Mister Angry
>
> Then it got to be more at night-time. It was really Mister Angry. Clenched fists, rising knees, and really writhing about, and we thought, 'Right, he's got colic.' So I went to get some medication and I spoke to the health visitor and we all agreed that he'd got colic. The time of day that it was...

While many suggestions were made as to the nature and cause of colic, it was striking how certain some parents would be of their information or perspective.

> Colic is trapped wind. Wind that they can't get rid of. Screaming, isn't it? Drawing their legs up.

> Tummy ache! That's all it is. It's like when we have eaten a big meal and we've not eaten anything all day and your stomach cramps up.

> Trapped wind in the tummy. And it comes on in the middle of the night and they've got tummy-ache.

Such association of colic with trapped gas was very common, and perhaps represents the common lay perspective. Other explanations included association with vomiting, extreme hunger and simply crying at specific times of the day (notably the early evening). Experience with other children played a part, too.

Perhaps the most striking aspect of this attempt to associate the crying with a meaningful diagnosis was the disappointment and disbelief
brought about when the colic continued beyond the expected point of
recovery. There was considerable confusion about the meaning of
'three months colic'.

> 3.15: Which three months for 'three-months colic?'

> Well, I thought the colic was sorted out because he'd
> passed three months old and I'd been using the Infacol,
> but then it came back.

> It would be interesting to see if when he's [rapid calcula-
> tion] five months if it stops. If, like, that's his three months
> colic. People said, 'It's just colic and it will only last three
> months.' Everybody said that.

> She had just come up to about three months, so that
> seemed like a clear pointer that this was just colic. She'd
> been crying really badly before that, too, though.

For some this indicated a syndrome which should have resolved by
the time the baby was three months old. Others understood the syndrome to indicate that it would last for three months and then pass.
Still others thought that the three months indicated the supposed time
at which the crying ought to begin. The importance of folk lore and lay
belief in parental attitudes towards colic can hardly be exaggerated, and
the misconceptions illuminated in the quotes above form part of the
problem presented to health professionals by exasperated parents of
persistently crying babies. In fact, the meaning expressed by Illingworth
(1954) in his seminal paper was that the symptoms of colic would
usually resolve by the age of three months.
One facet that united all, however, was the disillusionment when
the supposed time limit proved to be false.

> 3.16: April and Tania – The crying just goes on and on

> Even with the solid food April was just the same. It's just
> gradually, very gradually gone away, like faded, over until
> she was about nine or 10 months. That 12 weeks thing
> for the colic is a load of crap. It just goes on and on.

> ... And it doesn't necessarily go away after three months, either. Tania suffered with it for a year. I mean, where do they get this 12 weeks from? What a load of rubbish. I've never heard such a load of tosh in all my life. Twelve weeks! And then they say that breast-fed babies don't get colic. That is a load of rubbish!

Having clung to one of the supposed three months rules many parents felt desperately disappointed and even betrayed when the crying continued. A telephone survey of the crying behaviour of 662 children in Germany revealed that of the 21% of babies reported to have cried excessively in the first three months of life almost 40% continued to exhibit the same problem for significantly longer (Wurmser et al 2001).

Not surprisingly, then, in view of the most accepted definition of colic, this as a diagnosis often failed (eventually) to satisfy parents in their quest to find a cause and a cure for the crying. They were, indeed, left with only a semantic gain. They now had professional recognition that they were coping with a baby who cried excessively for an unidentified reason. Searching for the diagnosis could not stop, however, once colic had been addressed with whatever degree of success.

Search, hope and disappointment

Something that almost all the parents readily recognised in their own behaviour was that, despite all the signs that a cause and a cure were unlikely to be found, they could not stop looking for potential causes and remedies. The search for the diagnosis was not continuous but was an intermittent activity with periods of agitation and quiescence. It appeared that the activity of seeking a cause for the crying would continue until all known avenues had been exhausted. Then a feeling of having tried everything, with nothing left to consider, would set in and life would settle down (relatively) with a general acceptance that this was the way things were going to remain for an indefinite period. While not approximating to normal life, since the baby would continue to cry and disrupt all activity, there was some degree of psychological fatalism and acceptance. Then another stimulus would appear. It might be a magazine article, a television programme, or simply someone else with another idea, and the frenzied search for a diagnosis and a cure would begin again, only to end in disappointment, frustration and despondency.

After trying the usual medications without effect Susan had undertaken an expensive course in learning to perform baby massage and had great hopes that this would soothe Malachy. Unfortunately, this, too, failed to stop the crying.

3.17: Malachy – Well that was nice but it didn't work

I did feel a desperate need to do something. But in my case, I wasn't getting the result that I wanted, so I didn't feel the relief that I was looking for. It was nice doing the massage, but I didn't get much out of it, really. I was doing it for a purpose and it didn't help that purpose.

Sarah and Richard's investment in cranial osteopathic treatment for Patrick seemed at first to have the desired effect. However, as the weeks wore on, it became clear that this, too, had failed, reluctant though Sarah was to admit this at the time.

3.18: Patrick – Another disappointing treatment

I suppose, really, because I knew that nobody could help him, because there was nothing, we thought we'd try it [osteopathy]. For the first treatment Patrick seemed to be better for two to three weeks. I don't really know whether he actually cried less or whether I just coped better, now. Richard thinks there was no difference at all, but, well... Like he says, I felt better about things. The second time we went, the crying seemed better just for a few days but then was as bad again. And the last time it didn't really have any effect at all that I could see. Not really, now that I'm honest about it. So that was a blow, another disappointment. As Richard says – an expensive disappointment.

Roisin painted a much more vivid picture of her disappointments which spanned some four or five months and which 'ruled her life'.

3.19: Scott – Bang goes another miracle cure

It's like the stuff they gave us yesterday. It's the first time he's had it, so now we're thinking, 'Right. He's had two lots. It's going to take two days to work. OK. We should see an improvement by three days.' And you build your life around it: 'We should see an improvement by... whenever.' So then you get disappointed. Constantly. The medicine we got on Thursday from the paediatrician: he actually said to us, 'You'll probably find that this is the miracle cure you've been waiting for.' Right. Comes rushing home. Gets to the chemist. Get it down him. Waited and

> waited. Then he started screaming, and he screamed even
> more. Bang goes your miracle cure. The doctor took it off
> us yesterday. There's another disappointment.

The sequence of trials and disappointments could lead to desperation and a willingness to try almost anything which promised a cure.

> You get to a stage where it's a shot in the dark. It's, like,
> people say, 'Have you tried this? Have you tried that?' and
> we would have tried anything, you know?

> If you said to try putting her to sleep upside down hanging from the chimney stack, you'd try it.

The psychological effect of repeated disappointment could, however, be considerable, particularly when parents already felt emotionally fragile. Resignation to simply having to cope and get along until the crying eventually stopped of its own accord at least brought stability, and any minor improvement could be considered to be a bonus. Unfulfilled hope, however, could damage the relative (and fairly minimal) peace of this acceptance.

> 3.20: No better off – and maybe worse.

> You try anything. If anybody can give you a bit of advice
> that you think you can use, anything at all, even just using
> a different teat for the bottle or whatever, you'll go out
> and buy it. Anything at all. You do it. Problem is, of
> course, none of it works and you're left no better off,
> maybe a bit poorer, and sometimes it may even seem
> worse than before. It, like, knocks you back when you
> build up your hopes and then it doesn't work.

Some parents remarked on the effect that this exerted on their readiness to accept that things had improved when they did. Being so ready to be let down again caused them not to dare to believe that the crying had reduced. It was usually a matter of a slowly dawning realisation that life had become a little easier; gradually, perhaps imperceptibly. Each minor improvement could not be accepted until sufficient time had passed to prove that it was more than a temporary respite.

Two respondents summarised the contrasting outlooks that illustrate the ambivalence of parents' responses to the crying and the absence of an explanation. Most participants experienced both perspectives at various times. One approach is a particularly functional perspective on the subject of searching for a diagnosis.

> People start calling it names of one sort or another, but to me it's really just crying. And most of the time I just think that whatever the cause is it's probably different every time, and a lot of the time there probably isn't a cause, really, anyway.

This realism may have resided within each of the participants, emerging from time to time as they exhausted the current range of possible causes. Far more time would be spent in searching for the diagnosis, however. Yet even during these prolonged periods there might be insight into the folly of their quest.

> I think that's probably where I got it wrong, though, or at least where I made it worse for myself. I couldn't stop trying to find the cause. I mean, you don't. You don't stop until... well, in my case until he'd grown out of it.

The superficiality of the 'recovery' from the drive to find the cause became evident in the conversation with Helen who was pregnant again and admitted:

> Doing it again makes you really think hard. I'm already looking for the cure before he's even born.

This speaks volumes of the intensity of the urge to discover the cause and establish a diagnosis and of the longevity of the effects on parents' lives of living with a crying baby.

Chapter 4
Effects of excessive crying

Some of the effects of excessive crying have been considered already, particularly those relating to infant feeding. Frequent changes of formula, early weaning, addition of noxious substances, and (most sadly) the abandoning of successful, established breast-feeding are all common results. It was also seen that efforts to analyse, assess, and intervene in cases of excessive crying can sometimes be confounded by the complexities of feeding problems and the baby's aberrant sleeping routines in association with excessive crying. Families, too, are often confused, and they use the issues of excessive crying, poor feeding, and problematic sleeping patterns interchangeably during discussions and consultations. Sometimes, a fog of confusion falls, and interventions are attempted without a clear link to the perceived problem. The problem and its effects often then persist unabated.

Long-term effects of excessive crying

One common reason for anxiety among parents was the thought that the crying would have long-term consequences for the baby, and, indeed, such matters have been the subject of a number of research studies. A few examples will have to serve here to demonstrate the point.

Excessive crying and asthma

It is a common myth that excessive crying in infancy leads to the development of asthma during childhood. Given that some cases of excessive crying might be related to cow's milk protein allergy, atopic disease might realistically be expected to be associated with an increased degree of crying. However, in a prospective follow-up study of 116 infants considered to be at high risk of atopic disease Kalliomäki et al (2001) found no difference in the total distress (all degrees of fussing and crying) between those who developed asthma and those who did not. Moreover, in a large prospective study (983 children enrolled at birth, of whom 9.2% were diagnosed with colic) Castro-Rodriguez et al (2001, 878) found 'no association between infantile colic and markers of atopy, asthma, allergic rhinitis, wheezing, or peak flow variability at any age'. Parents can be assured with confidence that excessive crying does not cause the development of childhood asthma.

Excessive crying and later emotional regulation

A common concern of parents is that excessive crying in infancy might lead to sustained problems of emotional regulation during childhood and beyond. Indeed, examples have been provided earlier in this book of just such an assertion on readily available Internet sites offering advice to parents. While there was some difference in some aspects of emotional behaviour in post-colic children at four years (although open to interpretation), in all other respects no significant differences were found between the post-colic group and a control group in a Swedish study by Canivet et al (2000). Neu and Robinson (2003) found no such correlation at all in their comparative study of six to eight-year-olds who had been previously identified as having or not having had infantile colic.

Excessive crying and maternal mental health

Another common assertion is that the mother's mental health may be irreversibly damaged by the process of coping with a baby who cries excessively. Allowing for the inevitability that all parents are affected and in some way changed by the process of parenthood, this position is again overstated and unnecessarily pessimistic. In a prospective cohort study of 856 mother–infant dyads, in which 6.4% of infants were declared to have suffered from colic, Clifford et al (2003) found no evidence to support the notion of lasting effects on maternal mental health.

Excessive crying and mother–infant relationship

The potential for excessive crying to provoke loss of bonding and the consequent increased risk of non-accidental injury must, of course, be of concern. Yet while many parents would recognise the danger of a sudden outburst of exasperation resulting in a hasty act ever to be regretted, this is a different matter to the notion of permanent or long-lasting problems in the mother–infant (or father–infant) relationship. As with many other suggested lasting effects of excessive crying this is, in fact, far more rare than might be thought. Barr (1998) analysed four follow-up studies of infants with prior colic to find that in only a small sub-set of families with additional pre-existing risk factors might a general 'persistent mother–infant distress syndrome' evolve. For the majority, however, the crying was seen to resolve spontaneously over time leaving no residual effect of relationship or attachment difficulties.

Wurmser et al (2001), in a large survey of 662 children in Germany (in which 21% were found to exhibit excessive crying or fussing in the first three months), noted firstly that the crying persisted for longer than three months in almost 40% of cases. However, only weak evidence was found of potentially persisting problems in the relationship between parents and infants. Moreover, in The Netherlands Van IJzendoorn and Hubbard (2000), replicating an earlier longitudinal study of infant crying, attachment, and maternal responsiveness demonstrated that mother–infant attachment at 15 months was unaffected by the crying. The overall result of this evidence is that persisting problems in infant–mother relationships are not a likely outcome of excessive crying.

Actual effects of the crying

Most people would be able to guess at some of the other effects that excessive infantile crying could exert upon family members. These ideas might well revolve, for example, around issues such as loss of sleep or problems with the baby's siblings. Issues like these can clearly be important for some families, but they may also be viewed as being symptomatic of a wider, more pervasive effect. Most participants in this study experienced disruption to almost every aspect of their individual and collective lives. Relationships between family members could be affected, social isolation could be experienced, and concern about the risks of non-accidental injury to the baby could lead to feelings of 'living on the edge'. Together with other factors this often resulted in feelings of guilt on the part of parents, a guilt which seemed to lurk in the background despite external reassurance and efforts to consider the situation rationally. No-one in the household escaped the influence of the baby's crying and all were affected in various ways. This was found by Raiha et al (2002) in Finland, too, in a study employing videotaping of interactions and applying standard assessment scales (though with a fairly small sample).

Disrupted lives and unrelenting demand

Babies that cry excessively often exhibit aberrant feeding patterns. They may refuse to feed when they are clearly hungry; they may refuse to be held; or they may simply cry during all efforts to feed them. The latter appeared to be the main problem for the families in this study.

4.1: Francis – Painting the Forth Bridge

The feeding makes coping with the crying more difficult.
You know, as well as crying anyway, he's feeding every
three hours. Particularly at night, by the time you've
changed him and fed him and brought him back it's been
an hour gone by. Like if you've started at one, it's two
o'clock when you've got back to bed, and at four o'clock
it's another turn.

In this case crying disrupted the feeding routine such that more time
could be spent in accomplishing the task than was left between feeds
for other activities. Engaging in this at two-hourly intervals was not
uncommon. Since all of the babies were putting on weight in a satisfactory manner and were also achieving developmental milestones, the
feeding regimes, however onerous or even bizarre, were generally effective, and this is the case with most such babies. However, the effect on
the parents was notable. Many parents will be aware of the demands
placed by feeding any newborn baby, but they would expect the situation to ease gradually. The problem is that this is simply not the case
with babies who cry excessively, and the disruption continues.

In a similar manner, sleeping patterns were reported to be an excessive problem. Parents were disappointed that their baby failed to fall
into the expected pattern of feeding, playing (or at least responding
pleasurably in some way) and sleeping. However, if the baby had simply remained awake but was quiet and content there would have been
no problem. The failure to sleep was problematic only because it was
accompanied by the persistent crying and screaming that affected other
parts of people's lives. This became particularly acute, of course, if the
disturbance continued through the night and the rest of the family was
unable to get sufficient rest. Susan and Alan, living in a small terraced
house with Malachy (11 months) and Eoin (7 years), for example,
could find no means of preventing everyone being kept awake at night
by the crying (including neighbours at times). Alan's work as a driver
was clearly affected, while Eoin was showing signs of being tired and
disruptive at school.

The issues compounded each other. A baby who had not slept
(because of crying) may be too agitated to feed, while feeling hungry
could prevent the baby relaxing sufficiently to sleep. The problems of
crying, not feeding, and not sleeping were, therefore, closely inter-
woven, but the root cause of the families' difficulties lay in the crying.
Feeding problems were generally the result of the baby's crying, while
failure to sleep became a problem only when the baby spent this

waking time crying. This is borne out in the literature, too. St James-Roberts et al (1996) found that 'persistent crying is intertwined with a less obvious, but potentially equally important, disturbance of sleeping'. Crying impinges on time that could be spent in sleep. The complexity of cause and effect relationships in crying, feeding and sleeping problems is noted by other researchers, too (Michelsson et al 1990). What is not left in doubt, however, is that the problem exerts a serious effect on the affected families. Tired, frustrated, and often worried, parents may experience a number of other effects that further reduce their quality of life and indicate the need for support.

Relationships – together, but apart

A feature of the experience of living with a crying baby that was common to everyone in this study was its effect on family relationships. The more serious problems tended to relate to the relationship between the parents, but more guilt was felt about difficulties caused with the baby's siblings.

The relationship between parents

One father summed up the general thrust of feelings by referring to a line from a Dire Straits song: 'It's like that line, isn't it? We say it's like that line from Dire Straits ... "You and me go parallel, together and apart." That's just what it's like.'

'Together but apart' was an expression that was consonant with the experience and perceptions of other families, too. Sarah and Richard, for example, noted the same effect, adding that efforts to takes turns or decisions for one to sacrifice free time or sleep for the other's benefit compounded this.

4.2: Sarah and Richard – Together but apart

Sarah: Yes. We've got to stop and make a conscious effort to say 'Look, I want to tell you about so and so that happened today.' You've really got to make a conscious effort to do that and talk about things. Or you try to do it last thing at night when you're both tired out and not really listening.

Richard: We've been prepared to sacrifice, to have that particularly hard time because the other one has

> been able to benefit. So, I've got to give some-
> thing up so that Sarah can do something. That
> means, of course, that I'll be with Patrick while
> she's off doing something else and vice versa, so
> you only get things done by being separate.
>
> Sarah: Meals in shifts, too. That's the usual thing, isn't
> it? One has their tea and the other one... [Peters
> out with a gesture towards the children.]

There were many other examples. One couple joined a video club expecting to spend time together in the evening watching a film after their baby had gone to sleep. Nine months later they had still not managed to watch a single film together because of the baby's crying. Helen had been used to keeping an hour or two free with her partner each evening but since Michael had cried so persistently this practice had ceased. 'I think our relationship suffered as a consequence,' she said. 'We're so stressed. We have no time together; no life.'

A different mother spoke at length and very openly about a specific effect on her relationship with her husband. Her story recounted details of the demise of the couple's sex life, with increasingly frequent arguments and irrationality, leading eventually to accusations of absence of concern and even infidelity. Lack of affection, lack of time, and lack of inclination added to a powerful formula for dismissing any possibility of an active love life and seriously threatened the marital relationship. Because of the crying, she asserted, 'It's a loveless marriage with a relationship that won't exist until the crying stops, if even then, and we argue about it all the time.'

Conflict between parents and between partners was expressed in other ways, too. For some this was not a major part of the problem, however, and Joanne was clear that, for her, the conflict was limited to occasional shouting matches about allocation of work. Claire, too, told me that she and her husband 'had their moments' but this never deteriorated into blazing rows. She put this down to his prolonged absence, especially at the times when she was most agitated about the crying. So, while she missed his support at the worst times, at least their separation prevented them turning upon each other. At other times, and for various families, the conflict can be characterised by particularly petty arguments.

4.3: That's what it does to you

> We argue about who's spent most time with him that day.
> Because it gets petty, very petty. Does it really matter that
> you had him for an hour extra or more than the other?

Out of a whole day. It's pathetic, really. But that's what it brings you to. And you can have a huge blazing row about it. Over one hour or half an hour. It's just... so petty. I tell you. It just shows what this crying brings you to. It just takes over so much. Any other time you'd laugh at someone having such a stupid argument, wouldn't you? But that's what the crying does to you.

This specific issue of the division of labour caused much resentment and many arguments. A lack of communication between partners was often very clearly a factor (and expressed as such by the participants), more so because it could lead to a misunderstanding of each other's role and the rigours of each other's daily life. Studies involving families with chronically ill children (Bradford 1997, Sabbeth and Leventhal 1984) have found these factors to be common, too. Another exchange between Sarah and Richard expressed this clearly.

4.4: Well, what do you expect me to do?

Sarah: He keeps saying to me, 'Oh, there's something wrong with him.' And I say, 'Well, I've taken him to the doctor and they've checked him out and they say there's nothing wrong.' And it's got to the stage where I've said, 'Look, you take him!' I feel like he expects me to do more, but there is nothing I can do. We aren't on the same wavelength.

Richard: I'm almost saying, 'That's not good enough.' I'm out at work all day, so I can't take him, and I'm sure there is something to be found and that she's being fobbed off. I suppose I mean, 'Don't come out of the doctor's until they've given you an appropriate answer...'

Sarah   I know he doesn't mean it like that, but I keep thinking, 'What do you want me to do?' I feel that he thinks that because I'm at home I should be doing something to sort it out. But I don't know what I can do.

Julie also perceived this pressure from her husband to do more. She knew that breast milk would be the best for her baby, but her husband's expectations of her in this activity only added resentment to the stress she experienced in trying to cope with Nicola, and finally she stopped breast-feeding and gave Nicola formula milk instead. Occasionally, the resentment could take over completely, and two mothers told of deliberately (if without forethought) injuring their husbands – one by stabbing with scissors. These appeared to be extreme cases, but they are indicative of the level of stress prompted by the crying.

Siblings

All of the families with previous children were in agreement that the siblings of a crying baby suffer as a consequence. Claire, the mother of Fleur and Jason, thought this but added a cautionary note that other stimuli might be causing the aberrant behaviour demonstrated by siblings.

> 4.5: Jason – Not everything is caused by the crying
>
> I think he is affected by the crying, but there are lots of other things going on at the same time, so you don't know whether it's the crying or something else that's making him behave in a certain way. It might be just his age. He's growing up. He's got to put up with things at school. There's the usual clashes when he wants something he can't have.

This salutary note serves as a reminder that normal issues can easily become obscured by the depth of focus on problematic issues. Despite this, it was clear that concern about other children added to parents' difficulties. Sometimes it is self-evident to parents that older children suffer from lack of attention. As Sarah indicated in the first interview:

> Oh, well, if the baby's crying, his big brother doesn't get any attention at all. I find it difficult to concentrate on playing with him while the baby's screaming his head off. I feel a bit better about it now that the first one has started going to nursery. At least he's getting some entertainment.

Concern about this lack of attention, mixed with a large dose of guilt, was also expressed by Tania's mother.

> 4.6: Tania – It's your fault!
>
> 'Poor old Tania's homework is going [indicates throwing over shoulder]. She's started shouting at us. [Imitates child's

voice] 'I didn't do my homework last night. It's your fault.'
You feel terrible. I've actually signed her homework book
sometimes without her doing it just to make her feel better. She's said, 'Just sign it' so she won't get into trouble.'

Bradford (1997) and Drotar and Crawford (1985) found such
changes in sibling behaviour and the resultant guilt felt by parents to
be very common in cases of chronic illness in children – children, of
course, who often require more time and attention from their parents,
as do crying babies. More than one mother admitted that her first child
was smacked more often while the baby's crying was at its worst. This
was linked to an increase in demanding behaviour on the elder child's
part: a change noticed by others, too. Elaine was finding that James
(aged four) was increasingly vying for his mother's attention.

If Harry starts crying when I'm trying to feed him, James
will go and do something that he knows he shouldn't do.
He'll start throwing clothes around or something. I suppose he's trying to get my attention. He's upset by the
crying. Sometimes he shows it by getting upset; sometimes by doing things that he knows he shouldn't do.'

This sort of behaviour exemplified the evidence which could be
observed at first hand in the study. Zach, aged three, had become
annoyed at having to wait for his mother's attention while she dealt
with the baby. He had already had a temper tantrum and had been rep-
rimanded for throwing food on the floor, and finally he picked up one
of the tape-recorders and threw it across the room. Such outright
expressions of frustration and anger were commonplace and appeared
only to add to the general difficulty of attending to competing demands
on the parents' time. What was of more concern to parents was the less
noticeable, covert reactions sometimes to be seen among siblings of
crying babies. Sarah remarked on a tendency which she had noticed in
her son, Francis (aged three).

4.7: Francis – Mum doesn't know what she's doing

Sometimes when Patrick's having a really bad screaming
do he [Francis] goes really quiet. He'll come and sit on the
floor near me: silent. He's done that a few times now. I
don't know what's going on with him. I think it does affect
him, really. Deep down it does register. There's something,

you know? It's like he's thinking, 'My Mum's not shutting
him up. She looks like she doesn't know what she's doing.'
I wish I knew what was going on in his head.'

Parents usually required little stimulus to identify causes for guilt within themselves. Feelings that 'a good mother' would cope and know what to do to stop the crying were particularly common, and this was an example of such reactions. Concern about the sibling's needs and the inability to attend to these adequately or in good time compounded the guilt already felt at being unable to stop the crying.

Social isolation

Feelings of social isolation are an understandable and realistic response to the situation faced by parents whose baby cries incessantly, and such perceptions were openly expressed by participants in this study. Michael had cried uncontrollably from two weeks after birth until about five months.

> 4.8: Michael – I couldn't take him anywhere

> I mean, I didn't go anywhere. I didn't feel I could go any-
> where. I didn't go shopping. I didn't go to see friends. I
> didn't go for walks. I didn't do anything. Everything just
> completely stopped. I think the strongest effect was that I
> felt really socially isolated. I couldn't take him anywhere.
> Certainly the social isolation thing was really significant.
> And it was more profound than you might think. I couldn't
> see any end to it. I mean, it was three months solid when I
> couldn't go out. That's when it was at its worst.

Rachel's mother, Eileen, reported a similar experience, with Rachel's father, Phil, adding that even though he went to work each day, between arriving home from work and leaving again the next day he felt trapped in the same isolation. Weekends were the same.

> I mean, what did we do last weekend? Nothing. And the
> weekend before? Nothing. And you can go as far back as
> you like for months: it will be the same answer. And that's
> not through lack of things to do or places to go. You just
> can't go anywhere or do anything when you've got a
> baby like this.

While the feelings associated with this restriction on respondents' own activity were commonly characterised by frustration and despondency, guilt was added when the effect on siblings was considered. This was felt acutely by Roisin, now coping with her second crying baby, and confirmed by Tania.

4.9: Tania – Missing out

But then, Tania [the six-year-old sibling] doesn't get to go out like we did before. We used to go out every Sunday lunch to a pub where there was a play area and a garden. We used to do all sorts of things at the weekend as a family and for her. I'd take her shopping with me. But now, because of the way he is we don't go anywhere. We daren't take him out, so she misses out.

Part of the problem appeared to be that normal sources of support and relief of pressure became unavailable. Helen had enjoyed the mutual support and friendship of other women at ante-natal classes, groups and clinics, but found this avenue closed when dealing with a crying baby.

4.10: What's that woman doing with that poor baby?

There was just no way I could go. He would just scream the whole two hours, while all the other babies were laughy-gurgly. It meant that (a) I got nothing out of it because I was unable to sit and talk to people: I was just pacing up and down trying to calm him down, and (b) there was the fact that, well, my perception that all those people would be looking at him and thinking, 'What are they doing with him? What is that woman trying to do to that poor child?'

Such perceptions of the disapproving judgement of others were widespread, and there was a noticeable association with perceptions of gender expectations. Both mothers and fathers felt that other people were at least implicitly criticising them for poor parenting, and sometimes the criticism was explicit.

You get paranoid. 'What's that woman doing to that baby?' You can hear them saying it. You know what they're thinking. You can see it in the looks they give.

All people say to you is, 'Ahhh, look at that baby. He's all upset.' You don't need that. You know he's upset. 'Why aren't you doing something about it?' That's the message they give. And sometimes they even say it. It doesn't make you want to go back.

We tried to tell each other not to let them put us off. But they did. You know: 'What are they doing with that child?' or 'You'd think she would do something: give her a bottle or whatever.'

We were always uncomfortable whenever we were out with her. People were always staring. This time you could see them talking about us. I was embarrassed, and maybe angry, too. Angry at them for doing that. You wanted to run away from them, didn't you [to wife]? I wanted to go and give them a talking to or worse.

The foray into the normal world even simply for shopping would often result in the hurried acquisition of vital items from the shopping list and a hasty retreat to the car and return home. What had begun as a social occasion would quickly deteriorate into an unpleasant and stressful task, not to be repeated until absolutely necessary.

This was not universally the result of such events, however. Stacy, who had found the courage to go shopping with a friend, each taking their babies, encountered the familiar response from on-lookers.

4.11: Oh, God! Let me go home!

We used to go walking around the shops and she used to be continuously screaming her head off. And I used to be thinking, 'Oh, God, let me go home.' But my friend could just happily carry on shopping. All I wanted to do was to get into somewhere under cover. Back to the car or something. She would just ignore it all.

At first it seemed that this had made a significant difference to her experience of shopping, but her explanation continued to reveal that in some ways her friend's insistence on ignoring the stares and the comments had served only to heighten her own anxiety and stress. She felt compelled to continue but could not adopt her friend's acceptance and bold approach. For her the ordeal was extended not resolved.

Another mother, Julie, with two children and additional experience of child-minding, had learned to ignore the staring and muttering, but she could not cope when people commented directly to her about the crying.

4.12: Snapping point

It was really more if somebody said something to me. If it was just me walking round with them and she was crying, I'd just hold my head up and think, 'I'm not even going to think what people are thinking.' But when they started saying things and giving me advice, that's when I got wound up. I was walking round Ikea. All these people started saying, 'Hungry baby. Hungry baby.' I just flipped. I said, 'Look! She's not hungry. I've just fed her. Now keep your nose out!' I went away and thought I was really awful, but I couldn't help it. You know? I mean everybody was so full of ideas.

Elaine, who clearly seemed to take the crying in her stride most of the time, partly, perhaps, because Harry was her second crying baby. Yet even she felt the same external pressures when out in public. Her specific problem related to breast-feeding her baby. The expected 'normal' restriction on her freedom from breast-feeding was augmented by increased frequency and lack of any longer interval between feeds during the night. The reason for this was the baby's habitual crying which defeated all attempts to establish a routine of a satisfying feed followed by a substantial period of sleep. Every episode of feeding would be punctuated by attacks of inconsolable screaming. Determined, at first, to pursue a normal life incorporating the normality of feeding her baby, she would attempt to shop in her habitual manner, but the baby's crying would so disturb other mothers and babies in infant feeding rooms that eventually she gave up and went home to feed Harry. So the isolation imposed by comments of strangers was not universal, and was experienced in differing degrees by individuals, but there remained a widespread reluctance to venture into public places such as shopping malls with a crying baby on anything other than specific missions and for the briefest possible visit.

Aborting visits and expeditions was commonly reported. One mother recalled leaving work-related social functions on three separate occasions because the baby's crying was so disruptive, others remembered numerous family outings spent retiring from the main party to relieve the stress on other adults and children of the crying, and some noted an inevitable reluctance of friends to keep in touch. Feelings of frustration often accompanied the embarrassment and anxiety provoked by these experiences. Even visits to friends and family resulted in similar outcomes and could be equally (if not more) stigmatising and constraining.

Visits from others to the home tended not to work out, while visits by the family to others fared no better, and parents felt reluctant to impose the problem onto others. This was often matched by a degree of resentment that other parents were not affected in the same way, and the feeling of isolation was sometimes exacerbated by the apparent normality and tranquillity of others' lives.

> It affected me at home as well. I mean, when people came round I couldn't have a conversation with them because he just wouldn't stop crying.

> We just refuse to go anywhere. We are falling out with people over it because we won't take him out. We don't take him anywhere on a weekend because nobody wants a screaming baby in the house.

> We just realised that although other people who had had babies at the same time as us were beginning to get some normality back into their lives and go out and so on, we simply couldn't.

One of the more telling aspects of this problem was families' inability to accept help when it was offered. Sometimes this would be a matter of fearing that the volunteer would be unable to cope. Other difficulties would relate to the parents' reluctance to burden friends or family with such an intractable problem. Often there would be expressions of feelings of duty relating to carrying the burden themselves. In any case, the value of such a break from the baby is questionable.

4.13: I wouldn't do that to my worst enemy

> I had a friend who offered to come round while I went into town or somewhere, but there was absolutely no way I could have someone baby-sitting him because he would just scream. No way. In fact his paternal grandmother came for a couple of hours while we went to get him registered. I left her a range of potential options, but of course nothing worked, and when we got back after a couple of hours she left. We didn't see her again for two months.   (Helen)

> I would rather stay here and cope with it myself than go somewhere and say, 'Help!' Because they've got kids of their own. They don't need that. But my friend... offered to have him all night on Friday. I said, 'You can't. You've got three kids, all under five.' She said, 'I can cope with one sleepless night.' I said, 'I couldn't do it to you.' She's offered to help. But you can't do it. I mean. She doesn't know him that well. It would probably upset him more.   (Roisin)

> People have offered. My auntie has offered to have him all
> day Saturday so we can take [sibling] out and do what we
> want. Do some shopping or whatever. But I have to say to
> her, 'Oh, the whole time we were out I'd be thinking, what
> is he doing to her? Does she want to throw him out of the
> window?' You know? And she says, 'Oh, I'd cope. You
> have it every day. I can cope for one day.' But you just think
> that I wouldn't do that to my worst enemy.   (Joyce)

In all, parents often felt trapped in a paradox. They would feel guilty for leaving the baby with someone else, but they felt a desperate need (both practically and psychologically) for a break and some space in which to achieve normal, mundane, everyday tasks. At least in some cases, parents were not only aware of the nature of the problem of social isolation, but also had some insight into potential solutions (even though they had been unable to effect these personally). Of course, being forced to face the traumas of venturing out with a crying baby may, of necessity, break the physical aspect of social isolation but it is no guarantee that the psychological aspect of isolation is addressed. Parents could still 'feel alone in a crowd', shunned and ostracised by those who felt they could manage the baby better and blamed the parents for ignorance or lack of commitment. Nevertheless, having a companion who would share the burden could offer a way out for some, going some way towards breaking the isolation imposed by the baby's crying. Helen remembered the walks that she had taken with her baby, Michael, accompanied by her health visitor.

4.14: Someone to share the burden

> When she came we would go for a walk with the pram and
> she would come with us. He would be screaming but it
> didn't seem to put her off. That helped. That boosted me.
> Psychologically that boosted me. Just when I was feeling
> most isolated she would come and listen and be shouted at.

This apparent therapeutic effect will be addressed in more detail in a later chapter.

Once again, the similarities between parents with crying babies and those with a child suffering a chronic illness seem quite extraordinary. The unexpected occurrence of the problem; the drawn-out period of trying to establish a diagnosis and secure effective treatment; the reluctance to accept the impossibility of a cure; and common effects of social isolation, self-recrimination and stress which are commonly found in chronic illness are often also to be found in excessive crying. Such factors are discussed at length by Dale (1997) and Bradford (1997) with regard to children with chronic illness, and they make interesting reading for any health professional involved in supporting parents with enduring problems in their children.

Desperate tiredness

It takes little imagination to conclude that crying babies cause loss of sleep for families, yet even this obvious problem is more complex than might be thought.

4.15: What's the hardest thing to cope with?

'It's got to be lack of sleep,' answered Mike, nodding his head vigorously. 'You can't cope if you're not getting enough sleep. That's when it really gets on top of you. And it pressures you, too.'

I'm finding that the longer this goes on the harder it is to sleep. I go to bed and lay there thinking, I'm so tired but I can't go to sleep. I just can't go to sleep, and I'm so tired. I can't switch off. I'm thinking, 'Well, I could just be doing this or that while I've the chance.' I find it very difficult to switch off, even when I get the chance.

Melanie said, 'If I've fed him at 11 and I've gone to bed at one, and I've fed him at four and I've got to bed at six, and he's up at seven, and then I've got both kids all day. Well, the first day I can cope, but by the second day I'm pretty much past it. And, you know, it goes on a lot longer than just two days.'

It just went on and on. There was no sign of it getting any better. Every week we'd say, 'We can't manage another week like this.' But another week would pass and we were all still here. Still alive if maybe not quite as sane...

The important part of such comments from parents is not simply that lack of sleep was a problem but that the problem could grow to have an excessively forceful effect on life, provoking stress and eventually ill-health. Most parents expressed concern about the extent of the physical and psychological effects of the lack of sleep, particularly as the repetitive nature of the disturbed nights exerted a cumulative effect.

Some, like Helen, charted the number of hours spent crying each day (although this included a range of intensity). 'I thought I might be exaggerating how bad it was. But I wasn't. One day it was 18 hours; 18 hours of crying in one day!' Roisin, meanwhile, reported that 'Anyone can cope with a crying baby if they sleep at night. He cries 24 hours a day. So, it's not like we get any let-up. We don't get any breaks.' Clearly, Roisin was not suggesting that Scott cried continuously every minute of every hour of every day. It might well be that, if asked, her estimate of the total number of hours that Scott spent crying each day would be grossly inaccurate. However, this is not the key issue. The problem in her experience (and that of other families) was the absence of any reliable and lengthy period of time each day when the baby would not cry. This disruptive effect of the unpredictability of the crying featured in the findings of St James-Roberts et al (1996), too.

The most obvious response to the chronic loss of sleep might appear to be for partners to take turns to accept a broken night, but this often meets with limited success. Peter recommended that sharing the load was the crucial issue.

> Trying to get one of you to get a good night's sleep is really important. One of you has to put up with it for that night and the other gets some sleep. If one of you can get some sleep, and if you can see that the other one is getting past it, then you take the baby away from them. Even though you're still tired, you take it away from the one who's had enough.

However, Roisin explained the problem, 'We take it in turns, one night each. But that doesn't crack it because you're still disturbed. You can still hear him. I can hear every wriggle.' An alternative perspective was offered by some parents in which sharing the task of comforting the baby and lending mutual support were important features. Sarah described this.

> We've both tended to bring him downstairs rather than have him crying. So one tends to warm the bottle up while the other comes in here and tries to keep him quiet. So we're both getting up and both being disturbed. But you couldn't sleep through it anyway.

This was not always an agreed strategy, but it could meet the differing needs of each parent in some cases. For Eileen and Phil there was a disagreement about the value of both parents getting out of bed to their baby Rachel.

4.16: It works for me!

Phil: Yeah. It could be quite annoying sometimes. I'd get up at four in the morning to comfort Rachel.

Eileen: [Laughing] And I'd be sitting here beside him, giving orders.

Phil: I'd think I'm giving Eileen some sort of night's sleep by coming down here and pacing the floor. The next thing she's stood at the door. Well, what's the point of that?

Eileen: I just needed to be here, to see what was... I know it used to exasperate Phil sometimes, but it made a difference to me just not to have to physically deal with her. I could sit with a cup of coffee in my hands and watch. That was enough for me. It was almost like a break.

In the attempt to understand the effect of the crying on the family it can be all too easy to forget that each parent may have different responses to the crying, be affected in different ways, and need differing support to find relief.

Elaine, who was breast-feeding Harry, provided a further perspective on the complex, multifactorial nature of the effect of the crying when the whole family is taken into account. She, Robert (her husband), and James (their first son) were all disturbed by Harry's crying every night. There was no possibility of taking turns with the feeding (apart from changing the baby) to allow for respite, and neither was there any other way to escape from the crying.

My husband is always very tired. James [four-year-old sibling] often wakes in the night as well with all the noise, and Robert goes into James. And then when Harry [15 weeks old] is crying so much during the night anyway, we're all awake. So in the morning Robert is just really jaded. He's just always tired. He goes to work tired.

For Melanie, whose baby April cried from two weeks old to nine months, the support that she desperately needed dissolved because of the night-time crying. At the time that the crying was at its worst she was living with her family and later at the house of her partner's mother (while he was working away).

4.17: Melanie – Feeling forced to move away from support

A lot of my family, though, from when she was little, and when I was at his Mum's, they couldn't cope with her crying during the night. Because they couldn't get any sleep themselves. Also, they were all working, so there were no volunteers for help. I could see that they had just had enough of it. That's when I moved here. Alone.

The effect of the crying on the rest of the (extended) family was such as to drive Melanie away from the support that she probably needed.

Other family members would confirm the effect upon them. Susan and Alan, the parents of Malachy (11 months) and Eoin (7 years), the children's grandmother (Muriel) and aunt (Diane) would often be together in a small council house which seemed very cramped. Five adults, two children, a dog and a cat made for a noisy and claustrophobic atmosphere. Even with just the parents and two children, when the baby cried unceasingly for hours during the night there could be no evading the noise and the stress. Diane had explained her role in supporting her sister in caring for Malachy. She would call in each day and spend time with them, taking turns to soothe the baby and do other jobs around the house. The time would come, however, on some days when she finally could take no more and would find an excuse to leave and go home for a while. Muriel, although she would usually see the day through, admitted to similar feelings of rising tension and a desire to flee. The support remained, but the stress increased. During the night the parents coped alone. Obviously, coping with crying through the night was especially trying, and could lead to increasing fatigue.

Much of this suggests that crying at night is mostly the root of the problem for parents, but this is not always the case. Certainly, lack of sleep made life more difficult for affected parents, but this is not to say that crying only in the daytime is not a serious problem. Indeed, this pattern of excessive crying can present its own problems. Melanie was unequivocal about the problem of daytime crying.

What! I didn't have any time at all. I couldn't get anything done. I never had any time of my own. It was all trying to stop her crying, and trying to feed her or play with her or whatever. I never got over it.

Other parents, too, asserted without any hesitation that the frequency of the crying was the key factor. Given the option, they would have preferred to cope with crying '...over a longer period but less often. Because in between, if it's night-time you can get some sleep. If it's during the day you can get on with things. It's more a matter of disruption than anything else.' A significant respite either during the night or during the day would have made a serious difference to the parents. The relentless nature of the crying prevented any return to normal activity, reinforcing instead the primacy of the crying in the family's life.

Unfortunately, such relief was likely to be short-lived. However brief the respite from the crying, the time was usually then snatched to catch up on household tasks.

4.18: What can I get done? (I should be relaxing.)

My childminder had him for an extra couple of hours on Saturday. So I came back and thought, "What can I do? Get my head down or catch up on the housework?" And the housework wins. Every time. I got the hoovering done. I got the polishing done. I got two lots of washing done. I polished the bedroom which hadn't been done for months. By the time I've finished there was no time left to rest: I just went and picked him up again.' (Roisin)

Even when other people find time to take Yvonne away and I'm supposed to have a rest, I sit here and I think, 'I could just be cleaning the bathroom, or whatever.' I do stuff like that. I know I shouldn't do it. I know I should be sitting down and relaxing. But I can't do it. I can't leave stuff lying around. I seem to do everything when she finally goes to sleep or when someone takes her for an hour. But that's really the time when I should be relaxing. (Stacy)

Life had become a blur of perpetual hurrying: a constant readiness to snatch the briefest of moments to achieve some routine task that has been delayed until the opportunity arises. Even these moments could be interrupted and tasks simply had to be completed while the baby cried uncontrollably. Richard, whose two sons had both cried excessively, recalls how things had been at the peak of the problem with the younger of the two.

4.19: All this to do, and he's just screaming away.

There'd be jobs to do around the house. If we hadn't done any cleaning for ages we'd just have to forget about it because we were occupied by one or the other of the children, more usually Patrick. If he was quiet, pretty rare, or feeding, the other would be mixing up bottles or something. It was, like... You'd go out to work. Rush out. He [elder son] goes to nursery two days so that's a rush. Come in at night and the first thing is to make up bottles while they have their tea, and then we have to try to find some time for our tea. Then it's bedtime for one and another bottle for the other... And all of this is going on while he's screaming away and you're trying to pacify him. While he's screaming away, you're at your wits' end. You've done all you can but he won't settle and sleep. All these other things to do, and he's just screaming away...

This hustle to get things done while simultaneously trying to soothe a baby and attend to the needs of the rest of the family, all within the context of chronic tiredness and absence of any expectation that tomorrow might be different took its inevitable toll on the parents. Eileen felt this haste and its consequent effect of disorientation particularly acutely.

4.20: Eileen – What day is it?

I'm just so tired. Simple as that. I'm just really bad at trying to remember the things that I've got to do. I wasn't like that before. You coming here tonight. I must have said to you [husband] about four times, 'Did I say six o'clock? Did I say half past six? Maybe it's not tonight. Maybe it's tomorrow night. Maybe it's next week.' ... Or if he got a phone call and it was really important, I might remember two days later. Or I make a shopping list and go without it. I wouldn't ever have dreamed of even making a shopping list before. I'm just a wreck. I need to catch up about three days' worth of sleep, but I can't.

Another effect of the excessive crying involved a tendency for parents (or more commonly, mothers) to question their own actions and to ask the question, 'It's not me, is it?' Such feelings of being 'helpless and guilty in the face of such alarming and uncontrollable behaviour in young and vulnerable babies' were also found by St James-Roberts et al

(1996). Perceptions of being compared to (apparently) more competent mothers were common, although a simple self-assessment of worth and ability as a mother regardless of others' ability often resulted in a negative self-portrait. Despite any evidence that their parenting skills were lacking (indeed, the literature suggests that often they were likely to be more skilled than other parents) many mothers concluded that they must bear the blame for the baby's crying. Even the most confident would find their faith shaken as the crying continued day after day. Elaine, who appeared to be coping best of all the parents in the study, was not immune to this self-doubt, and she introduced a connection between this and gender expectations. Her thoughts gave voice to the turmoil of care, concern, confidence and doubt.

> 4.21: Elaine – A good mother would do better
>
> I wonder quite often... I don't think it's something that I'm doing wrong. It's just that he's had a bad start. Still, I can't give up trying to make it better: looking to see if I could do something better. For as long as he carries on crying I can't help feeling that I ought to be trying something else. I'm sure it's all to do with being a mother. A mother ought to be able to make things better. But you can't. There's nothing to be done. I do know it, inside. But that doesn't stop the guilt. Yes: it's guilt. Even though you know you've done all you can, you always feel like your best clearly isn't good enough and you need to try harder. It's not my fault ... but there's always that niggling doubt.

The obvious (although undeserved) guilt and self-recrimination felt particularly by mothers, though shared at least to an extent by some of the fathers in the study, indicated that reassurance from external sources that the parents were not to blame was clearly a vital issue. Aside from the unpleasantness of such self-doubt, the lowering of self-esteem and damage to the confidence of the parents served to increase the overall stress they experienced, in turn reducing their ability to look ahead to better times and a normal life with the baby.

Living on the edge and non-accidental injury

Other effects on people's health, borne out once again by Bradford (1997), included missing meals or eating irregularly or late at night; a vicious circle of contracting colds, aches and pains and other minor illnesses; irrational anxiety about work problems; inability to keep minor issues of daily life in proportion; and emotional lability.

Regarding the last of these, Joanne, suddenly clutching Zach (her three-year-old first son) to her, and with her mother nodding vigorously in agreement, recalled a particular incident with her baby of 10 weeks and Zach. Her mother had been on holiday for two weeks, and she had missed the support. Both children had been especially demanding seemingly all day long, and finally she succumbed to the pressure.

4.22: It takes you to the edge.

I just sat down and shouted to Zach, 'Can you not just stop for a minute?' And I was bawling my eyes out, and that made him cry. Seeing me losing it was just upsetting him more. I think you get used to a level, even though it's a very low level. Then, when you get too much aches and pains, and the pressure is too much, it takes you over the edge. And it might not take much to send you over that edge, either.

This is a particularly graphic way of considering the situation of coping with excessive crying: an image of existing on a plateau of exhaustion and grinding effort until an event (foreseen or not) pushes the parent too far and that parent loses control and self-restraint.

Sometimes the response to the crying would include only mild annoyance or frustration. 'You can get quite wound up and frustrated,' said Claire. 'Why can't you just be happy for a while?' Elaine admitted to thinking, 'Well, if I'm holding you, walking around with you, and I can't stop you crying, why am I bothering with you at all? Why don't I just leave you to it? It's almost like, "Stuff you Jack!"' The frustration could be linked to other feelings. 'The effect on my partner was different,' began Helen. 'For him it was, like, "Ahhh! Why is this happening?" You know? More like angry or frustrated. He had a feeling of "Why have we ended up with this baby?"' There were clearly also other times when the reaction to the crying was more pronounced. Peter, talking of his second crying baby, noted the need to recognise and remember that the baby was too young to be deliberately obtuse and frustrating. Despite the perceived provocation parents may need purposefully to focus on staying in control, remaining patient, and keeping a reign on their temper. Others supported this, remembering numerous occasions when they had to recognise their mounting frustration and failing patience and take active steps not to lose control.

Helen vividly remembered habitually shaking and screaming at her husband when he arrived home from work, 'thrusting this crying bundle into his face' and metaphorically washing her hands of the problem for a while. This was clearly an adaptive behaviour: a deliberate strategy to deflect anger from the baby and to secure a release of tension. It was a foreseeable event at a predictable time, understood in its nature by both partners, and essentially self-limiting. It could only occur once each day. The effect was immediate: the payoff worth the price.

There was general agreement among participants that excessive infantile crying holds a quality which makes it especially difficult to bear. Marianne remarked that even some three months after her baby's crying had abated she could not bear to listen to another baby crying. If the crying continued for more than a few minutes she found herself becoming tense and irritable and simply had to get away from the sound quickly. This was only one of several examples of comments that suggested that the experience may be buried only very shallowly in parents' minds, ready to be awakened by a variety of stimuli.

Two other facets of parental responses to the crying give cause for concern. The first was reports that there was no pleasure in the baby, and the second an admission of an absence of bonding. Each, of course, is well-established as a contributing factor to the incidence of child abuse. A number of studies has indicated that excessive crying alone may increase the risk of non-accidental injury (Frodi 1985, Barr 1990, Crowe and Zeskind 1992). When added to other established factors such as absence of bonding and prematurity the risk increases significantly. Admittedly, not every family reported difficulties in this area. Julie was quick to point out:

> I love her. I love her more than anything in this world. I think I've a thicker bond with her than I ever did with Lucy [3 years old]. I know it's probably not normal, but I never once had an awful feeling for her.

Others had experiences which were common to many parents but which were exacerbated by also having to cope with a crying baby. Joanne, for example, explained about her need to restrict touching of Mark for the first five weeks because of his prematurity and his need to be left to conserve his energy. Then, when she was able to handle him she had to go back to work. Mark's grandmother undertook most of his care for some time so that his mother felt an absence of bonding for months, and was unable to respond effectively to his crying. There were more explicit expressions of difficulty in bonding.

4.23: Susan – Just physical care

No smile, no. It was either he was asleep or he was in pain. Nothing else. And we thought, 'This can't be right.' People say, 'Oh, they're adorable, babies of that age.' But to me it was just the worst time. The worst four months. We didn't have a relationship with him. It was just physical care. No pleasure. Nothing. He didn't feel like part of the family.

Helen and Marianne were even more unequivocal about their negative feelings, particularly about the experience of breast-feeding.

4.24: No fun – just a screaming lump

I was expecting all that stuff that people say about feeding being a wonderful time, and the closeness and all that. I didn't feel any of it. There was no fun in it at all. Not an ounce of pleasure from the whole business. We had no bonding moments because he was just screaming the whole time. It didn't have any impact at that time, but in other circumstances those would be the sorts of things that would lead you to throw your child across the room, because you haven't been able to form any bond... I know my partner looks back on it all and sees it as more negative than I do.   (Helen)

I think it has had a lasting impact, really. Personally, I don't think I really bonded with her until she was about five months... for a combination of reasons. But people talk about this eternal thing that happens at birth. It didn't happen for me then. I was expecting it to kick in at some point soon and it didn't. There was just this screaming lump, and I never felt that, 'I would die for my child' thing for a long time. By six months it was there.   (Marianne)

Many parents spoke openly about the possibility of non-accidental injury: either its likelihood, or their fear of being suspected. One father suggested, 'We've all had those thoughts at some stage when we're tired and you could throw them out of the window.' Another mother agreed, 'Not a lot of people would like to mention it but it does happen. You do get fed up, and it could happen.' An experienced mother remarked that her husband was often worried about her being alone at home with the baby. 'I mean, he has actually said that he's expected to come home and actually find me saying, "Sorry, I've done something terrible." And it frightens him.'

Speaking about the real possibility of harming their baby in a moment of crisis and extreme provocation is an uncomfortable, distressing experience for most caring parents, yet several parents in the study found the courage to do so in a very frank exchange. The words of Eileen and Mike paint a vivid picture.

4.25: How close to the edge am I?

Eileen: After I'd been with her all day it would get to the point where I just wanted to shake her. I was in such a state when he got home that I was inconsolable, wasn't I? And she was crying and I was crying. I think it's just that you get to a point where you think, 'What am I going to do?' ... It frightened me so much that I was out of my wits, really. The damage I could have done. 'Am I safe to be with her on my own?' was what I was thinking. 'What about tomorrow? What sort of state will I get into tomorrow?'

Mike: Had it been 10% worse, would I have done it? And you don't, but suppose it were 10 or 20% worse. Would I do it then? It's scary. It's, like, 'How close to the edge am I? Was I miles away or was I already right on the edge?' That's really frightening.

Eileen: I think it would frighten me that if I did do it and the damage was done... The fact that I could actually... It was being out of control, almost. I just had her, and I went [indicating agitated behaviour and desperately looking around for something]. Put her down! And it's like, 'Oh, my God!' The sudden realisation. The shock that I got.

Such moving accounts emphasise that, at least for the families that participated in this study, excessive crying exerted profound effects on the family. Almost every aspect of life was affected by the crying, and no-one in the family escaped its influence. Sleep, work, meals and social events were all interrupted or curtailed. Relationships between parents became strained and siblings suffered, too. In addition to physical and mental exhaustion, two major effects were to be noted.

The first was that of social isolation. This had both physical and psychological manifestations; isolation sometimes being caused by the reactions of others to the crying, but at other times being self-imposed through reluctance or inability to indulge in social activity or to accept help. The second effect related to what participants referred to as 'living on the edge'. This anxiety-provoking phenomenon resulted from the cumulative effects of exhausting physical and emotional effort, increasing frustration, guilt at being unable to soothe the baby, self-confessed lack of bonding, and isolation. At its worst, living on the edge was characterised by a repetitive alternation between approaching and withdrawing from a perceived point where control was lost and the baby was at risk of harm. Although these fears had not been realised for any of the families in the study the anxiety provoked by the possibility of an incident caused great distress. The disruption to life brought about by excessive crying was too intense to be tolerated without attempts to resolve the problem. These attempts are discussed in a later chapter.

Chapter 5
Parents' efforts to cope

Having considered the practical problems and effects associated with having a baby who cries excessively and the more active, animated (and ultimately disappointing) part of the cycle of hope, active search for a diagnosis, and repeated disappointment, this chapter turns to the way that families cope from day to day and the factors that help with coping. Parents are likely to feel a compelling need to respond actively to the problematic crying, and some of their more radical responses may be maladaptive. There is evidence that all manner of strategies are tried in an effort to improve the situation, some of these potentially dangerous or even fatal. Van der Wal et al (1998) identified the following strategies:

- Shaking
- Administration of laxatives
- Slapping
- Administration of sedatives
- Smothering
- Administration of painkillers
- Swaddling
- Placing the baby to sleep prone
- Stopping breast-feeding
- Admonishing

Sometimes a degree of relief is obtained, although often short-lived and sometimes at a price that may be only marginally acceptable.

A number of theoretical perspectives are espoused on the subject of coping, including physiological, psychoanalytical and interactionist contributions. The latter, attributed largely to Lazarus and Folkman (1984), fits best philosophically and practically with the focus of this book. It represents coping as a process characterised by efforts to survive and manage stressful stimuli and events. More recent work based on these thoughts defines coping as 'a self-regulatory process that is purposeful and intentional. By coping, the individual or family system reduces or prevents the responses that normally occur under stress' (Hymovich and Hagopian 1992, 171). Although criticised by Carver et al (1989) as being over-simplified, coping is divided by Lazarus and Folkman (1984) into problem-focused coping, which predominates when positive action to address the stimulus can be contemplated, and emotional coping, which is more often a feature when it is believed that a stressor simply has to be endured. An example of this would be the specific coping strategies exhibited by parents in a study of sick infants requiring home cardio-respiratory monitoring for an average of six months (Stevens 1994). Both of these are to be found in the participants in this study. Issues that relate mostly to problem-focused coping predominate, but it is foolish (if not impossible) always to separate these two aspects of coping activities (Carver et al 1989). Elements of emotional coping are also readily visible.

Specific coping strategies

The need to be organised and to enforce a routine for the baby was expressed by several participants.

5.1: Planning to keep ahead – just.

I like to be organised before he goes to work because if not I feel like I can't cope with the day… At least I've got a chance to keep on top of everything. But if we start off already behind I know I'm not going to catch up. (Sarah)

If you knew, say, that on Wednesday afternoon you'd have an hour without distraction you could plan what best to do with the time. For example, washing isn't a problem. You can throw everything in the washer and the dryer easily enough. But ironing can be really difficult to arrange. Now if I knew that I was going to have an hour's grace tomorrow afternoon, I'd have all the washing done and a pile of ironing ready to dive into.   (Claire)

This feeling of a lack of slack in the system, with no tolerance for lost time and an automatic penalty for slackening the pace, was a standard feature for others as well as Sarah. In addition to the serious perception of 'living on the edge' with the deeply significant consequences of realisation of its potential, there were, perhaps, many smaller event horizons which held the less serious threat of a day of disorganisation and rushing in vain to catch up. Being able to plan ahead for the day was important, even if to secure only an hour's allowance for undertaking other tasks. The problem with this, of course, was that the desired hour's grace could not usually be foreseen. Nevertheless, when it was possible, being able to plan ahead even on such mundane matters promoted some notions of being in control again.

Their experience with Rachel's crying led Phil and Eileen to aim for better planning all round before their next child.

> I think what made things worse was the notoriously bad planning on our part. We moved here in the March. We had her in the October. I'm going on a college course in September. I've got a full-time job. We had a baby, and a house that needed decorating all in one fell swoop. I think we must have been in self-destruct mode. I think if we were to do it again, with the benefit of hindsight, we'd organise things a hell of a lot better. We'd say 'Right. The only thing that I've got to focus on is work and Rachel, and nothing else for the next 12 months.' But then, if you plan for your children you'll never find the right time. (Phil)

There is, of course, nothing unusual about a young couple moving into a house that needs decorating eight months before their first baby is born, and neither are additional demands from work a surprising event. Perhaps this was another manifestation of the tendency for parents to blame themselves for the crying and of the need to attribute the problematic situation to some tangible cause. Nevertheless, planning ahead to reduce the effect of particular events is recognised by Carver et al (1989) to be a common part of active, problem-focused coping.

5.2: Establishing a routine – with varying success

> I could never get into a routine with her... because she was cat-napping all day and when she woke up she was just screaming all the time... Now that she's getting older her stomach's getting a bit easier, but she's still not got a sleeping routine or anything.   (Melanie)

> We do the same thing every night. She has her tea; then she has a bath; then a cup of hot chocolate or whatever;

then she goes to bed. We've got the routine down to a
fine art. She just isn't sleeping.   (Stacy)

Peter, the father of Andrew, Gail and John, was enthusiastic about
the need to keep to a routine for the baby including feeding, bathing
and sleeping, recognising that otherwise additional periods of crying
during the night were especially likely. Even though the crying
remained excessive and difficult, the enforcement of a routine helped
to effect some slight improvement and constituted a positive action in
tackling the problem. Melanie was in agreement with the importance
of routine but had failed completely in her efforts to achieve this with
her baby, April. Seeing no result from her efforts, she gained nothing in
physical or psychological terms. Stacy and James, too, were struggling
with finding a balance between causing Yvonne to be especially tired
before bedtime and establishing a normal feeding, bathing and sleeping
routine. Whatever they tried appeared not to work. Such disappointments can easily lead to what Carver et al (1989) term 'behavioural
disengagement' in which there is a reduction in the motivation and
energy to resist the stressor, and other unassociated goals may also be
abandoned. Establishing a routine may help with coping as long as a
positive result, however small, can be observed. The minimal nature of
the changes in the baby's behaviour that were considered to be an
achievement by some parents suggests that the benefit may be drawn
more from a minor moral victory rather than from a significant change
in the crying.
    While establishing a routine for the baby was generally viewed as a
desirable aim for crying babies (as for any other baby), the tedium of
the routine for parents could be problematic. Speaking about her husband returning from work to be confronted with a crying baby, Joanne
concluded:

Well, it is hard, when they've been out at work all day and
then they have to come home and cope, but I think the
other side of the coin is that I've been here all day and my
shift is no easier. And I think just doing something different makes the biggest difference.

5.3: The relief – and guilt – of a respite

That little break was really important, I think probably one
of the most important things was my friend coming round
to give me those few precious, and, it seemed, very brief

> moments to myself. That little bit of relief and the chance
> to catch your breath. That mattered.   (Helen)

> If you have somebody who can take them out for you,
> maybe give you an hour in the day where you can get
> work done, I think that would help. It's when you haven't
> got any time to yourself that it gets really difficult. Even
> every other day would help.   (Claire)

Opportunities for distraction from the focus on the baby's crying and occasional relief from the daily grind and routine were prized by participants. These were seen as islands of normality in the sea of chaos that formed the greater part of life. The most common strategy was to be separated from the baby for some period of time. For Peter this occurred when he went to work. 'It's not until I can stop and have five minutes to myself... that I remember about the problems.' Richard, too, found relief from the crying in going to work, but suffered feelings of guilt in return: 'You're out of the house and driving to work: it's like a respite from the crying.' By comparison, for Sarah this was usually a matter of leaving Patrick with his father or grandparents while she went to the supermarket with Patrick's elder brother. While this may not appear to be much of a break, Sarah assured me, 'I still feel the relief. I mean, it is so much easier when you can get away, in a lot of ways.' Helen felt the same way. She had a friend who would take Michael out to the park for an hour or so while she attended to the housework that had built up – a treat that she described as a few brief moments to herself. The break provided by relatives and friends was used by Roisin, too, for completing housework, although the opportunity was valued nonetheless. 'She put him in the pram and off she went for an hour and it was absolutely ace. A full hour without Scott. I managed to get some cleaning done and all sorts. For an hour.' Claire, by comparison, could only muse on what would have helped since she had no family close enough to take Fleur for a while.

Not everyone wants the children taken away for a while, however, as Julie explained while reflecting upon her mother's idea of helping.

5.4: Julie – Help *me* to cope

> She'd think that she would take the kids out of the way
> and that would help, but that wasn't what I wanted. I
> wanted to be with the kids myself... I want her to stay with
> me and spend some time with me and help me... Help
> would be to spend time with me and the kids. I wanted to
> cope with the problem not be separated from it.

Julie's approach may have been illustrative of another aspect of coping: 'mental disengagement' (Carver et al 1989). While distraction from the problem may be adaptive sometimes, it can prevent or delay the coping activities which more directly address the difficulties in the family's life. Julie wanted to face up to her problems and find solutions or means to control them. She sought 'instrumental social support' (Carver et al 1989) in the form of the company of a helper. The varying attitudes towards offers to remove the baby for a while are indicative that any effective attempt to intervene on either a lay or professional level would have to address the individual needs of the family. Certainly, there is a fundamental need of parents to be listened to and for others to try to understand the individual circumstances of that family. Here was a mother struggling to gain the understanding of her own mother.

5.5: Claire – the value of distraction

Often I think she was better being with other people, maybe with something else going on, some distraction. Or maybe it was just that I was distracted and there wasn't any difference in her. It just seemed that way. Perhaps it's just easier when your mind is taken off the crying for a while and you're not so focused on her.

Another means of securing relief was to dilute the problem. Sarah found attending a toddler group to be effective in reducing the load of attending to the needs of both Patrick and his three-year-old brother Francis. Although she did not get away from the baby, having other mothers around and pooling resources to care for a group of children (some of whom would be much less demanding) was a significant aid. A similar story was told by Stacy about days spent at her mother's house with many other family members. With so many adults and other children to provide distractions Stacy could relax her constant vigilance and attention to Yvonne and 'switch off' for a while. This was experienced by Claire, too. In all, then, time out from the crying can occur in a number of forms and does not necessarily involve physical distancing from the infant. However brief the period provided for a break from attending to the crying, it is valued and makes a practical difference to coping.

5.6: Leave him to cry – he'll soon stop

Joanne: You see, my neighbour next door, she's expecting hers at the end of June and she says 'Oh, leave him. Leave him to cry. He'll soon get out of it.'

Vivienne: Some people do. One of my friends waited years for a baby and she left her for hours to cry. I don't know how she could bear to listen to the baby. She's just that sort of person.

Joanne: I thought, 'Well, if that's the answer, I'll leave him for 25 minutes and if he does go off then that's the answer and I will leave him.' But you have no choice left. He's absolutely screaming his head off and I thought, 'I just can't do that to him.' It's not fair to him. I mean, it was just making him ill. He was coughing and spluttering and then he'd be sick. And I just thought, 'I'm not doing it.'

Leaving the baby to cry is commonly included in lists of advice for parents and is certainly part of lay knowledge. Peter declared himself to be 'a firm believer in letting the baby cry and see if they grow out of it'. However, Joanne and her mother, Vivienne, expressed more reservations. Peter had met this response before and had concluded that it was simply a matter of confidence and personality. 'They [the babies] can do it there next to me. I can switch off. That helps. Because if I know they're just whining away for attention and everything I can just switch off.' Although being sure that there was no reason for the baby to cry was an important factor, Peter recognised that there was also something about his own personality that allowed him to tolerate the sound of the baby screaming and crying. Downey and Bidder (1990) certainly found some very limited evidence of a sub-group of more neurotic mothers who were more prepared to leave the baby to cry, but, from their accounts, this would hardly apply to Vivienne's friend or to Peter.

The effectiveness of leaving the baby to cry was found to be variable among participants. Claire had tried this strategy a few times without success. 'I've tried leaving her to cry and she's cried and sobbed for an hour. I've done that and she gets into such a state and won't go to sleep.' Elaine, in contrast, found that 'sometimes he can't be calmed down and I end up just putting him down and leaving him to cry it out. And he does cry it out eventually. But at night I can't do that.' This was because of disturbing the rest of the family, particularly Harry's father and brother. Concern about disturbing the sleep of her school-age daughter was also a factor in Janet's reluctance to leave her baby to cry for too long. Flawed understanding of how to apply this strategy was also evident. 'We've tried it,' said Stacy, 'but you can't leave her for too long because she'll think we've gone out.' Leaving a baby to cry need not imply shutting the door and not returning until the crying has stopped. Most authorities advise parents to return to the baby at given periods (perhaps 15 minutes, for example), to let the baby know that someone is there, but not to pick the baby up and not to linger. There should be no suggestion of the baby suspecting complete abandonment. Nevertheless, even when an appropriate routine is followed the process can be deeply distressing. It may require persistence over weeks before a result is achieved, and there can be no guarantee that a positive change will be noted. The guilt that pervades the experience of living with excessive crying also plays a part. The remorse which accompanied Eileen's efforts appeared to upset her deeply. 'I've left her to cry from two months for two hours. But when you go to look at her to check she's still OK, the look that she gives you... I feel so guilty.'

5.7: Helen – Yes, I've tried that, too.

I tried all sorts of noises. Someone said that white noise was supposed to be effective for some reason so I tried it. I tried the hair-drier, the hoover, the washing machine, all sorts of music: loud. Sometimes he would actually stop crying, but not go to sleep or settle. He'd just lie there looking stunned. I don't suppose it did his ears any good, but at the time I thought that anything that stopped him screaming had got to be giving his voice a rest. The crying didn't actually stop, but it would be less... It had to be loud. It was wild what I tried. I tape-recorded the hoover and extractor fan. I played a rain tape. A babbling brook tape. He wasn't into the soothing stuff. It had to be loud and raucous.

All the usual strategies practised widely among parents without particular problems of crying were, of course, pursued. Putting the baby to sleep in a separate room; judicious use of dummies; carrying; rocking; pushing in a pram; and so on occasionally provided a little relief, but these interludes were either short-lived or infrequent. Less common possibilities were also considered though with no more success. Helen (5.7), along with several others, had explored the possibilities of noise as a pacifier. Apart from these and leaving the baby to cry only one other strategy proved to be relatively frequently attempted. This was driving around in a car with the baby.

5.8: Balancing the risks – driving under the influence of a crying baby

Is that a good solution: to be driving around going nowhere in particular when you're already tired? No. It isn't. Not at all. But we did quite a bit of it, really. In the afternoons I used to just stick him in the car and go driving. You know: not anywhere. Just driving. It's the relief – partly from the noise, partly from knowing that I was doing something. He just seemed so distressed and finally he was getting some sleep that I knew he must need. He was, almost at peace for a while. If I can stop him crying then it's obviously better for him because he's not distressed and I'm not distressed. (Helen)

To get him to sleep they take him out every night in the car. People do that, but there again, if you're that tired you shouldn't be driving a car. People do, I know they do. They take them out in the middle of the night to get them to sleep. You can't concentrate when you're that tired. It's the baby's life as well as your own that you're risking. You could nod off at the wheel. Fortunately, I've only had to do it twice. (Peter)

Helen described the list of schemes that she had tried in an effort to stop the crying, all with the same result: 'No difference. The only thing that actually stopped him crying was driving in the car. That's the only thing. Everything else failed. Everything.' She continued to explain, however, using one particular example, that 'five seconds after the car stopped moving, before the engine was turned off, he started again. So you couldn't even just have the engine on: you had to actually go somewhere.' Vestibular stimulation, the most likely explanation for the effect of driving in a car on crying, relies upon changes in velocity and direction, so this would account for Helen's observations. Claire experienced the same reaction with Fleur, who would go to sleep almost instantly in the car but would wake up immediately and start crying again as soon as the car stopped. Janet and Peter were the most explicit in their recognition of the risks involved in driving while exhausted and suffering from chronic shortage of sleep. Admitting that he had succumbed to the temptation himself on two occasions, Peter told me about his sister's approach with her son and acknowledged the risks involved.

So even though the relief was temporary, time-consuming, and perhaps dangerous, Helen felt that it was therapeutic in a practical sense and provided a precious respite for both of them, albeit brief. Joanne, too, recounted that Mark would sometimes sleep in the car, waking up as soon as the car stopped. She added that, apart from the cost of petrol (half-jokingly), this strategy was flawed in that she had another child to consider who had needs that could not be met while she was driving around in the car.

Other activities were further examples of the acceptable risks that families would take in order to secure some brief respite from the crying. Weaning the baby early was advised by professionals in some cases but most families resisted this until the baby was at least three months old. Even this, though, was acknowledged as a compromise between the ideal of not weaning before the baby was four months old and trying to improve the situation for the family. Other admissions of inadvisable behaviour were recounted.

5.9: Driven to desperate decisions

It happened by accident. He was crying and crying and crying: it was like an hour and a half. And in the end it went quiet and I looked in and his face was on its side but his body was on its front. He'd swung his knees over and he was on his bent knees. And that was the night that he slept for 10 hours. I never normally allow him to sleep prone. I always put him to sleep on his side. The soul-searching and self-recrimination that went on after that. Talk about feeling guilty.

Janet and Peter remembered having their baby in bed with them.

Peter: I've gone to sleep with him laying on my chest and just holding him. I know people tell you that you're not supposed to do it: you're not supposed to have them in your bed because you might roll over...

Janet: You do it.

Peter: If it means having some sleep, you do it. Put him in bed next to you and cuddle up.

The mother in 5.9 who allowed her baby to sleep prone felt driven by despair to accept what she recognised as unwise and inadvisable behaviour. She was well aware of the national 'Back to sleep' campaign, and knew of the increased risk of cot death when infants sleep in a prone position, but for one night a calculated risk was taken and never repeated. Many other examples can readily be elicited, but these should suffice to indicate that when the crying reaches a peak and parents' ability to cope is at its lowest, some risks may be deemed acceptable in order to achieve some rest and regain control of the situation.

5.10: A vital lesson – Look after yourself

I think in some ways it's being able to relieve how you feel: being able to talk about it. Releasing those feelings is important. If you bottle it up it's worse. Perhaps you don't look after yourself well; or you become moody. Then it's going to be harder to cope with it. (Claire)

In fact, I think if there's one lesson that I've learned for next time, or should I say, this time, it is to look after myself more. To see my needs more. I won't be as obsessive about breast-feeding this time. (Elaine)

I know I'm not a super-mum, and I wouldn't want to be a super-mum, but if I could just have not got so stressed out, if I could just have taken it more in my stride and perhaps let people help more. That would have been better. Maybe not to blame myself so much. (Julie)

As parents reached a point where they were resigned to living with the crying until it eventually subsided (or in one case where the crying had stopped some months before), it was not uncommon for them to reflect on their own health and how they would act differently should they need to cope with excessive crying again. Sarah, in the first interview, told me of the need for parents to make a conscious effort to look after themselves and each other and to find time for this. Several mothers recommended that parents should pay particular attention to their psychological needs, often reflecting on what they would do differently with their next baby. Reviewing their own expectations of themselves was part of the focus of this reflection.

Even though it may have been recognised late in the experience, the importance of emotional coping was evident. Perhaps the mothers could be wise only after the event, being so focused on, and dedicated to the crying before this. Nevertheless, the potential for an external agent to intervene and promote parents' reflection upon their own needs required investigation.

The role of the family in support

5.11: Helen – Having someone to scream at

If nothing else he was someone to scream at. That's really what it was. You know? 'Aaaahh!' [Imitating shaking someone and screaming at them] 'I can't do this!' Even just when you've had a day of it and he comes home and you thrust this crying bundle into his face and say, 'Here! You can have him for a while.' It helps to let the pressure off.

It is noticeable throughout this study that parents relied heavily firstly upon each other and then on their immediate family to survive the experience of living with excessive crying. There was agreement that coping alone would be extremely difficult if not impossible. One mother 'barely survived' the two weeks when her own mother was away on holiday. Her husband worked long hours away from home and spent many weekends (and five full weeks each year) with the Territorial Army, so her mother was her main and almost only support. Stacy was equally pessimistic about managing alone. 'Well, I'm sure that it would be a lot harder to cope if I was on my own. A lot harder... If you were by yourself you just couldn't do it. You'd just have it constantly.' This was certainly borne out by Claire who felt particularly isolated and recognised both physical and psychological problems in being alone with the baby. Melanie was also in no doubt about the necessity of support. 'I suppose having someone to help you was important. I couldn't have managed if I didn't have someone to help me. You know, his mum and then Mike.' In fact she had been alone for a few weeks and her situation then had been at its worst. 'Well, I only got this house when she was six months old, and I was on my own then. That's when it was worst. From then until a couple of months ago I was on my own. It was really bad.'

Sharing the load seemed to be the most important practical factor in the mutual support felt by parents. Some of the practical arrangements arrived at by parents in addressing the needs of their baby have been addressed earlier in discussing the disruption to life caused by excessive crying. The accounts of Sarah and Richard, Janet and Peter, and Phil and Eileen contain much vivid description of this. Sarah, for example, explained:

And, like, of a night – I try to catch up with jobs at night. So he'll [Richard] then spend the night playing with these

> two while I try to sort out what I didn't get done during
> the day.'

Apart from the practicalities of getting jobs done the parental part-
nership provided opportunities to release the pressure built up by the
constant crying (as witnessed by Helen in 5.11). Marianne supported
this feeling, remembering numerous occasions when she had also
been waiting at the door for Jessica's father, Geoff, to return from
work so that she could deposit the baby with him and go out of sight
and hearing to calm down again. It would appear that this facility to
vent feelings at a spouse is crucial to many situations of stress involving infants and older children. Gibson (1995) found clear indicators
that mothers resented and felt frustrated by their partners' lack of
attendance and participation in sharing the burden of concern and
physical care. Such paternal responses (even if due simply to absence
while at work) caused an increase in tension and a reduction in coping ability. In contrast, when fathers responded positively to the
mother's need for support and someone to shout at this provided
effective negative feedback to the mounting tension within the
mother (Whyte 1997, 8).

5.12: Julie – Both in it together

> We seemed to get through it better because we were
> both in it together than when Lucy was a baby. Then [with
> Lucy, now three years old] I just pushed him away totally.
> He wound me up... But with her [Nicola] we got on
> famously. Brilliant. He was so good. I can't fault him. I
> mean, we share everything: washing, ironing and every-
> thing. I think it brought us closer together if anything.
> [Sentence inaudible – children fighting and shouting]
> Yeah. I think it did. It brought us closer together because
> we were both in it together.'

A comparison was made by Julie between the infancy of her first and
second babies. She came to the conclusion that the second time had
proved more positive (and blamed herself for the problems with the first
child). In Claire's view, it was her separation from her husband for long
periods each day (and when Fleur exhibited most of her crying) that
prevented some potential problems in their relationship.

> I'm actually surprised that we don't argue more or get
> more upset with each other. Perhaps it's because she

sleeps OK at night and because he's not here when I'm most wound up. Now if he was here... You know, I can quite understand these stories you hear of women stabbing their husbands and throwing things at them...

Claire was especially confident and full of personal reserve. Perhaps her way was to cope alone. Most others, however, clung desperately to the support of their partner. Phil and Eileen summarised the importance of their mutual support and added an interesting perspective on the way in which this support might exert its beneficial effect.

5.13: Phil and Eileen – Sharing the burden

Phil: It was sharing the burden that made things easier and gave that illusion that she was better. But, in reality, I don't think she had actually changed... Psychologically it can be easier to cope with the situation if something affects us rather than Rachel. Definitely. The sharing of the burden is a good example, isn't it? That didn't make any difference to Rachel...

Eileen: Well, it did in that I was better at dealing with her when it was my turn.

Phil: Yeah, that's right. But the greatest effect was on us, though, wasn't it? Her care wasn't any different, substantially. Nothing different happened to her. It was us that were affected.

Peaks and troughs of coping

All families in the study experienced variations in their ability to remain positive and functional in the face of the crying. Claire, who more than most appeared to take the crying in her stride, acknowledged: 'I cope better at some times than at others, but I think I can keep it in perspective, maybe.' Others felt the variation more acutely, as expressed by Sarah. 'I think he seemed to improve a bit and when he improved I felt like I were getting up and feeling like I'd had enough sleep, but as soon as we had one night with just that little bit less sleep we seemed to go straight back down.'

5.14: Yvonne – Irregular cycles of crying

It's strange. We seem to go for about four weeks and be getting to the end of your tether, and then all of a sudden, for no reason, she'll just run out, she'll go to 10 o'clock, go to her own bed, and she'll sleep till, say, about half past six the next morning. She'll do that three nights on the trot and then scream for another few weeks. It's strange.

Life was characterised by peaks and troughs of coping. Just as with 'living on the edge', families would sink into a trough of barely coping with the next day or the next hour of the crying and then gradually (often imperceptibly) arise from the depths of despair onto a plateau of coping better and resuming a relatively settled life. This process would be repeated many times on an irregular basis until finally the crying abated and no further troughs of coping were experienced. One stimulus for this cycle of coping was that the baby's crying was not constant or consistent.

That the baby was not always crying and unpleasant might go unnoticed, giving a false sense that there were no normal periods in the baby's day. Sarah found difficulty in convincing Richard that Patrick did not cry all day long.

I say to him, 'Oh, no. He's been fine today. I've had him laughing and he's not been crying…' He doesn't cry all day. He might cry a lot, but when he's not crying he's quite a jolly little chap. I keep thinking, 'He isn't always like this.'

These periods of normality and absence of strife were usually infrequent and irregular, but Joanne noticed that finally a pattern was emerging in the crying. Mark had started sleeping for a six-hour stretch each day. This was a major improvement even though it was 'the wrong six hours', occurring during the evening and ending at two o'clock in the morning. It was just this sort of event which could stimulate recovery from a trough of coping. Other indicators were to be found of stimuli for this recovery which might be exploited to promote better coping. Phil, for example, remarked, 'I suppose the fact that you feel that things are not as bad as they were makes it not as bad as it was,' while Roisin had recognised the value of even minor achievements. 'We actually felt better after that. You know? A little victory. We've actually done something! And I actually felt good for a while.' Participants commonly had experienced uplifts of mood when small improvements in the crying had been noticed: a hint, perhaps, that there was a need for someone to capitalise on these opportunities: to reinforce the positive events and aspects of families' lives and to ensure that improvements in the crying and in life generally did not go unnoticed by parents.

Just as certain events and changes could lead to an increase in the level of coping, other occurrences or sets of circumstances could lead to a descent into a trough in coping. Elaine explained that it was an accumulation of negative experiences or factors that provoked a reduction in coping. This was the effect experienced by others, too, including Joanne.

5.15: Accumulated negative experiences

That's the sort of crying I can't cope with. When it's in the middle of the night and it might be waking the older one up when he's asleep, and my husband's having disturbed nights and going to work the next day, that's when I can't cope with it so well.   (Elaine)

If there's a lot of things need doing and you just can't get on, and it's getting desperate, and the end of the day, I find myself becoming really fraught and I just can't bear to listen to it any longer. And then Zach will start because he's wanting his tea at that time, or he's needing a sleep, or whatever else. I just find I'm coming to the end of my tether. And then you find one day's all right, and then following a good day you can cope, but two days together: by the end of the second day you're starting to think, 'I shouldn't be picking the baby up because I'm starting to just lose control.'   (Joanne)

The factors that could trigger a depression in coping ability were varied and unpredictable. It might be trivial events that finally broke the parents' resistance to adopting a gloomy outlook, and often the stimulus was not within the crying but part of the normal range of difficulties presented by everyday life. Such accumulation of difficulties, each in themselves perhaps of little significance, is often the cause of a gradual failure of coping for parents (Canam 1993). For parents in this study there appeared to be a point at which life switched from being characterised by control and coping to being dominated by the crying and associated problems. Gibson (1995) found such a turning point, too, which often implicated a conscious effort by parents to take control and move on with their lives.

As recounted in Chapter 3, life for the parents would cycle through stages of hope, active search for a diagnosis, despair and a period of relatively settled coping. This period was a function of coping, too, distinguished by resignation to the existence dictated by the problematic crying. Gibson (1995) found that mothers in her study also entered a period of resignation to their new situation through a process of self-reflection, eventually relinquishing their hopeless expectations of a cure. Perhaps due to having had insufficient time to indulge in such contemplation, the parents in this study showed little evidence of conscious self-reflection. Exceptionally, Marianne had realised rather earlier than most that a cure would not be forthcoming. For her the realisation that she would have to endure the problem occurred within a few weeks, and her explanation of coming to this realisation demonstrated admirable self-awareness and self-reflection. Most participants, however, found difficulty explaining this part of their lives, often concluding, as did Julie, that, 'You've just got to do it, haven't you? I really don't know how I got through it. I just don't know. I just muddled through, I think.' Claire expressed the same thought: 'It's just a matter of struggling to get by and get everything done. And that doesn't even mean doing things as well as you would really want them to be done. It's just coping. It's surviving.'

An element of adjustment to expectations, as suggested by Gibson (1995), was usually a feature of this phase. Julie recognised this.

> So a bad day with Lucy was probably when she cried for
> an hour, but a bad day now is when she's [Nicola] at it all
> day long. So now, with this whinginess: if this went on all
> day I'd have a really bad day. Otherwise it's a good day.

The decision that parents would simply have to cope with the crying for an indefinite period was sometimes thrust upon them by circumstances. Otherwise the conclusion was reached by parents themselves, as when Phil and Eileen gradually realised that endurance was the key and 'You've just basically got to sit it out'. On reflection, Helen was able to see that her health visitor had manipulated her survival through the troughs of coping and then continued to support her through the subsequent, more settled period.

5.16: Helen – hope in despair

> She used to come at least twice a week at one point.
> She'd say, 'You're doing really well. I don't know how I
> would cope with this. You're doing really well.' I'd think,
> 'I'm not, you know, it's just an act.' But looking back, that
> must have been a strategy that she used because I did
> cope and get through it.

The repeated disappointments and lapses into despondency appeared to create a barrier to recognising that the crying was finally resolving so that it could be some time before parents realised that their lives had improved. Such reluctance to allow hope of a resolution to enter the mind may be an adaptive response as a result of repeated episodes of failure: a protection against disappointment. However, part of survival when coping ability is at its lowest or when enduring the plateau of resignation, indeed the promise offered in times of coping better, is the knowledge that the crying must stop eventually. Even this, however, was not to be straightforward.

It will stop in time

It may seem obvious that excessive infantile crying is self-limiting; that the crying will stop eventually even without active intervention. For parents trying to cope with the problem when the crying is at its height, however, it can be difficult to accept this inevitability.

> 5.17: Elaine – Never mind tomorrow, what about tonight?
>
> It is difficult to even think about the future when you're coping with today and this feed, or its four o'clock in the morning and you've been woken up again. I think you go through periods of just not being able to see beyond today. That's when things are at their worst.

Some, perhaps simply more fortunate than others, had more reason to accept that the crying would stop in time. Sarah, for example, recognised that, 'In time they do grow and they improve, and they stop crying.' This was understood by Janet and Peter, too, who were able to draw on their experiences with two previous children who had cried excessively to know that 'they usually grow out of it within a couple of years... There's a good chance that he'll grow out of it. It will go away. It has done in John and no doubt it will in him [Andrew].'

> 5.18: Claire – Experience helps
>
> I think it helps having had another child. In a sense, you know you've been there, and you know it's going to get better. That ultimately she is going to get better than this. We will be able to get out and about without embarrassment and heartbreak and crying all the time.

Having experience with a previous child made a difference to Claire, who noted, too, that an important factor in achieving this reassuring state of mind was 'having that confidence, almost, that it is just a passing phase, and it will go away'. Roisin, a little sarcastically, suggested that Scott would get better despite the medical treatment.

5.19: Roisin – He'll get better in spite of everything

> I mean, we're doing all these tests, and taking him to the doctor's all the time, and giving him all these medicines. And what will happen is... he'll start to walk and all the problems and symptoms will disappear. It will go away. It will do, won't it? It will get better. No baby goes to school like this. They don't. But when you're coping with it day after day it makes it very hard to get by.

It was this confidence that was lacking in Julie who seemed to know probably almost subconsciously that the crying would stop but needed this reinforced by someone else. Speaking of the effect of the health visitor and what more could be done she remarked that: 'Maybe she could have rammed it home that it would stop eventually. I mean, I knew that she was gaining weight and there couldn't be too much wrong with her, but...' Elaine also admitted that she needed 'reminding that it will come right sometime'. This was mostly because of the immediate pressures of coping and the need to get through the next hour, the coming night, and so on.

Others had less cause to be positive about foreseeing an end to the crying. The most that Stacy could accept was that, 'I suppose I know that it will get better one day, but I don't feel like I can even think about it now.' Eileen felt no more positive than Stacy. 'I couldn't see any end to it. I mean, it was three months solid when I couldn't go out. That's when it was at its worst. It just went on and on. There was no sign of it getting any better.'

Helen was scathing of some professional intervention. 'I got sick of being told "It's just one of those things".' That was no use at all. Not helpful. I'd much rather be told that there is an end in sight: that it's not going to go on for ever.' Her impression of her health visitor was more positive. 'She said, "There are some babies who do this. Take heart: he'll grow out of it."' So what was wanted was an emphatic, unambiguous assertion that the crying would stop and life would return to normal.

For some, like Julie, the experience brought about a determination to understand and help her own children if they ever have a crying baby. 'Even when these are bigger, I'll never forget. And if they ever have one like this, I'll know exactly what they're going through. I'll help them. I'll never forget it.' This determination to help others in a similar situation was also one of the outcomes of the crying for Marianne. Her focus was a desire to help other mothers locally who were struggling with a crying baby. A final comment from Helen whose experience of coping with excessive crying resulted in a far less positive outlook speaks for itself.

5.20: Helen – What about the next one?

I haven't got that much positive to say about it, really, have I? But doing it again really makes you think hard. I'm already looking for the cure before he's born. I've stopped drinking caffeine. I'm already there looking for the potential cause. And do you know? When I see other mothers with tiny babies I have no coo-cooing instincts at all... Perhaps it's taken away my confidence. Perhaps it's taken away the magic. I thought it was all behind me, and we were getting on with life, and then this happens [Indicating new pregnancy].

This quietly-spoken moment of reflection illustrates the depth of the problem. That a pregnancy should begin in despair, anguish and perhaps resentment seems tragic. The experience of coping with excessive crying was clearly not a closed chapter in the lives of Michael's parents. The crying may have stopped but its effects were still to be found more than a year later, provoking anxiety and conflict.

Chapter 6
Interventions and support

With so little consensus on what causes excessive crying it is no surprise that there is equally little agreement on appropriate management or treatment. However, a considerable amount of study has focused on this aspect of the problem. A common practice involves testing a potential intervention for effectiveness in reducing crying and deducing from this (if it is successful) a probable cause for the crying. For example, if eliminating cow's milk protein from the diet reduces the amount of crying it might be the case that intolerance to cow's milk protein causes excessive crying. The inherent weakness in this approach is that causality is not necessarily established from a simple correlation, and a wide range of confounding variables may be introduced by the study method.

Although there are some notable exceptions, three approaches make up the bulk of the studies in this area: drug treatment, dietary modification, and maternal behavioural modification. A minority consider ways of helping parents to cope with the crying. One exception was Jayachandra (1988) who advocated removal of the parents from the crying baby for prolonged periods, and who provided explicit details of implementing corporal punishment for older children if such misbehaviour persisted.

Drug therapy involves the use of two main agents: dicyclamine hydrochloride and simethicone (referred to by many participants in this study by its proprietary name, Infacol). Illingworth (1959) provided some of the earliest evidence of the effectiveness of the former (an antimuscarinic or anticholinergic) preparation which reduces intestinal motility. Two further studies support this finding (Weissbluth et al 1984, Oggero et al 1994), but evidence, including that by Williams and Watkin-Jones (1984) and Myers et al (1997), demonstrates that the side effects of anticholinergics preclude their use in infants. These effects have been found to include respiratory collapse, coma and death. The work by Oggero et al is rather surprising in the light of this: the previously established effectiveness of a drug which is otherwise lethal seems hardly worth further investigation. Simethicone, an anti-foaming agent, is a safer drug but its effectiveness has been questioned. Danielsson and Hwang (1985) and Metcalf et al (1994) found simethicone to have no effect on excessive crying. However, its widespread use continues.

All the families in this study had tried colic drops, mostly Infacol. Most had used gripe water. A few had resorted to cranial osteopathy (discussed later). None had found a cure. What was apparent, however, was that the crying would often change during the period using medication but not subside.

6.1: The effect of colic drops

It was different, but the crying carried on. We would have a few evenings where it was easier solved and shorter in duration. So the crying changed, but it didn't go away.
(Elaine – using Infacol)

Well, they said to spend more time winding her, but I did. It would take me up to an hour to get one burp from her. They gave me colic drops, Infacol, gripe water and some other stuff for her stomach. None of it worked. Not at all. Not the drops or anything. She might have burped more but the crying carried on.   (Melanie)

This often had an unfortunate effect on the support from medical practitioners. Parents would find that the crying changed but remained, while GPs would assume that having diagnosed colic and provided the standard treatment the problem was cured. Joanne found that the colic drops made matters worse.

6.2: Mark – treated but not cured

… The first thing was that it was colic. So we dosed him up with the Infacol, and everything else, too, but it never had any effect. Nothing. Nothing at all. Then he started being sick. The crying didn't stop because of the drops, but he started being sick and crying more because of that… But then the doctors just automatically put it down as colic. And then, when you've treated them for it, that's gone away, so they think, 'Oh, that worked.' But the crying carries on. His crying was definitely different,

though. That 'angry' was really hard to cope with. That
really did my head in. Maybe that was the colic, rather
than just the crying.'

The notion that having diagnosed colic and prescribed Infacol the
problem was solved was one faced by Phil and Eileen, too. 'The GP,
well, really he just gave us a diagnosis of colic. The message was basically: "Go away and wait for it to pass off." He gave us the Infacol drops,
but they didn't do a damn thing.'

Sucrose, which has demonstrable analgesic effects in the newborn
and for many years was the main ingredient in gripe water mixtures,
was found effective in some cases by Markestadt (1997). However, this
finding has been criticised for being 'at variance with the experience of
UK practitioners. Children presenting with colic have frequently been
taking sucrose-containing gripe waters with no noticeable improvement' (Blumenthal 1997).

A number of practitioners recommend the use of herbal preparations. Weizman et al (1993) found herbal teas to be effective in
eliminating excessive crying in babies with colic, but serious methodological flaws and misrepresentation of the literature are indicated by
Barr (1993). Moreover, Cervisi et al (1991) warn that some herbal
preparations contain sufficient alcohol to exert a significant sedative
effect. Alcohol was formerly an ingredient in most gripe waters, too
(Illingworth and Timmins 1990).

Other treatments for colic fared no better. Claire had tried homoeopathic drops for Fleur after diagnosing colic.

6.3: Claire – Sorting out the colic doesn't stop the crying

The crying changed somehow, but it carried on. She was
crying, but it didn't sound quite as though she was in pain.
It was a mystery. Sorting the colic out did just that: it sorted the colic out. But it didn't stop the crying. Then I
suppose I was disappointed, but I had a sneaking suspicion
that it was too good to be true that everything would be
magically cured. In a way it didn't really surprise me that
the crying carried on. I did look for another explanation at
first, but then I settled down and just got on with it.

Dietary modification as a treatment relies upon the assumption of
some element of intolerance to cow's milk (or soya) preparations, and
much of this has been addressed when considering potential causes of

excessive crying. Perhaps the most rigorous study to date has been that by Forsyth (1989) which found that although elimination of cow's milk protein from the infant's diet improved the problem with crying initially, the effect was short lived and diminished steadily over time. Other efforts such as enriching milk formulae with fibre (Treem et al 1991) have met with no more success.

Studies investigating the effectiveness of practical supportive measures or counselling are often as equivocal in their net outcome as other approaches. Hunziker and Barr (1986) found that increased carrying reduced the amount of crying (but only in babies who cried normally), and Barr et al (1991) established that increased carrying had no effect in babies who were crying excessively with colic, a finding confirmed by St James-Roberts et al (1995). Elliott et al (1988) found gentle rocking to have no effect on babies who cried excessively, but McKenzie (1991) distinguished between stimulatory rocking and carrying and gentle rocking which is non-stimulatory, the latter being more effective in settling irritable infants. Huhtala et al (2000) were unable to show any significant benefit from either infant massage or the use of a crib vibrator. This is not to say, however, that each of these strategies is not worth trying or that parents will not feel some benefit – simply that no evidence could be found of any objective change in crying as a result.

An increasing number of studies address counselling or advice as an intervention, although with varying results. Pritchard (1986) provided anecdotal evidence of the success of practical parenting advice, and Kerr et al (1996) demonstrated that sleep problems can be positively affected by structured intervention with practical advice in a specialist clinic. A similar effect has been found in other studies through the application of a behavioural programme to increase sleeping (St James-Roberts et al 2001) and through the use of settling techniques combined with parent education and support (Don et al 2002). Counselling was held by Taubman (1984) to be more effective than other responses such as leaving the baby to cry, and structured behavioural management (by members of Cry-sis) was found by Wolke et al (1994) to be more effective than general support. Parkin et al (1993), however, found counselling to be no more effective than general supportive measures. Gillies (1987), accepting that little can be done to reduce the crying, found that practical advice and support could at least improve the parents' morale and self-esteem. Although the efficacy of supportive measures may remain uncertain, it would seem at least that the knowledge gained to date could safely guide practitioners in eliminating some of the dangerous soothing practices found by van der Wal et al (1998).

In the UK a specific service is offered for parents who are struggling to cope with a crying baby. Cry-sis offers a helpline from which parents can receive support locally from another parent who has experienced the same problem. In addition, checklists are available either in hard copy or from the website[1] – one for problematic infant crying generally, and another specifically for night-time crying. The general checklist is presented in question and answer form.

Is baby in pain?
• Check for illness or allergies with GP or health visitor
• Offer the breast, bottle or dummy
• Offer cooled boiled water, an infant colic remedy, eg Infacol, gripe water or baby herbal remedy. Try gentle massage of baby's tummy
• Try changing baby's position
• Pick baby up and walk about with him/her – a sling can be helpful
• Try gently rocking up and down

(From 'Crying baby? Guide to coping' Cry-sis)

For night-time crying a number of suggestions are listed:
• Rhythmic movement often settles babies. Rocking in a pram and gentle swinging in a crib can have a hypnotic effect. Baby slings can be useful as they provide continual movement plus the security of Mum or Dad.
• Soother tapes and devices may help babies fall asleep. A bedtime routine is a worthwhile investment for the future. This is best introduced as soon as possible with perhaps a warm bath before bedtime and a quiet feed and cuddle before sleep.

(From 'Crying baby? Guide to coping' Cry-sis)

Such practical advice is, of course, welcomed, but the most valuable contribution is probably a caring, understanding, non-judgemental friend on the telephone available to talk and listen at difficult times of the day.

While, as with this study, the role of counselling or some mode of support appears to have the potential for alleviating some of the distress experienced by families with a crying baby (Wikander 1995, Helseth 2002) little more can be held to be established with any degree of confidence with regard to treatment measures for excessive crying. A systematic review by Lucassen et al (1998) concludes that the best evidence to date is that a one-week trial of substituting cow's milk with hypoallergenic formula milk, together with behavioural interventions of general advice, reassurance, reduction in stimuli, and more effective soothing should form the mainstay of treatment. Such cautious advice is, perhaps, indicative of the state of knowledge of the causes and treatment of excessive crying.

A shot in the dark: cranial osteopathy

In addition to the GP and the health visitor, the contribution of one other practitioner was discussed by the participants in this study. Seven of the families were at least vaguely aware of the availability of cranial osteopathy. The Osteopaths Act 1993 established the General Osteopathic Council (GOsC), charging it with registration of practitioners, regulation of professional conduct and education, and development of the profession generally. Since May 2000 all practitioners must be registered, and the title of osteopath is protected by law in the UK. Information about this alternative approach to medical and psychological problems may be found on the website of the GOsC and other associated sites. The current GOsC website offers a factsheet which explains…

> The involuntary approach to osteopathic practice, sometimes referred to as 'cranial osteopathy' has developed from the discovery in the 1930s that small tolerances of movement exist within the human skull. From this, an approach to diagnosis and treatment has evolved in which the osteopath's highly trained sense of touch is used to identify and correct disturbances and limitations of tissue mobility, not only in and around the joints of the skull, but throughout the body. The technical approach used involves extremely gentle, but specifically applied adjustments to the movement of body tissues and is essentially a very safe method of diagnosis and treatment.
>
> http://www.osteopathy.org.uk (accessed 29.12.03)

As with most other treatments that parents discovered, no success was found with this therapy. Phil and Eileen paid for three sessions after finding that traditional medicine appeared to hold no hope for them.

6.4: Phil and Eileen – an apparent change, but not sustained

Eileen: It was available. OK, it was £20 a shot, but the GPs with traditional medicine didn't seem to be the solution.

Phil: If you get desperate enough you'll spend the money and try anything.

Eileen: Don't ask me what he did, but he massaged her head. Oh! And she was just in complete…..

> She went into a complete trance, didn't she? And I put her in my sling thinking she'd wake up. We walked round town for three hours: she didn't wake up. She was just completely and utterly relaxed. You could feel her little legs were limp. It lasted for three hours.

Phil: But there wasn't a lasting effect.

Eileen: No. Because obviously the first session there was no real change. We brought her back and she moaned and that. We went, and he basically said to us that it doesn't always work on the first time. We would need to repeat it. It didn't really have any effect on subsequent times, though.

Phil: Not at all. The effect was there, I suppose, after the first session, briefly. But it didn't last, and when we tried again it was useless.

So from three sessions and £60, a fairly standard fee according to the GOsC[2], Phil and Eileen found only three hours of relief. Sarah and Richard also tried three sessions with a cranial osteopath, seeking relief from Patrick's crying. They were only a little more successful than Phil and Eileen. Richard saw something of a psychological effect more on Sarah than on Patrick.

6.5: Sarah – maybe I felt better

Sarah: I've spent £75 on the visits.

Richard: And yet, he's certainly still crying just as much. We're spending this money and there hasn't been any noticeable improvement. I'm still woken up at four in the morning and he's screaming his head off. I think it's all had a lot more effect on you than on Patrick. But even so, even if it's complete trickery, I've seen the benefit in that you've relaxed. You've seen somebody doing something. And even if it hasn't had any direct effect on Patrick, it has psychologically on you.

Sarah: Umm. Well, I suppose it is true that for the first
            treatment he seemed better to me for two or
            three weeks. I don't really know whether he
            actually cried less or whether I just coped bet-
            ter, now. You think the nights were just the
            same as before, but... Well, like you say, I felt
            better about things. The second time we went,
            the crying seemed better for just a few days but
            then it was as bad again. And the last time it
            didn't really have any effect at all that I could
            see. Not really, now that I'm honest about it.

For the two families that tried this therapy, then, no significant benefit ensued. It would be inequitable, however, to criticise the
practitioners concerned for a success rate which was no worse than that
of traditional medicine in such cases. What was of more concern was
the manner of the presentation of the service. Among those who were
familiar with the existence of cranial osteopathy there was already some
belief about its role. The case of forceps delivery, for example, was quoted as an indication for such intervention. Claire had tried some
homoeopathic drops for Fleur's crying and colic but believed her case to
be not susceptible to osteopathy.

Some friends tried it. Their son had a forceps delivery and
they saw an osteopath with some degree of success. So I
was aware of it from them, but she was a normal delivery
and it never really occurred to me that osteopathy could
help. It's really for forceps deliveries, isn't it?

Helen had the same understanding.

Someone suggested cranial osteopathy, but that's really
for if it was a forceps delivery. A friend down the road
who had a six months old who would not sleep had been.
I think for the first session she thought he might be starting to sleep a little better, but after the second session and
all the others there was no difference at all. None.

Forceps delivery is indeed suggested by the GOsC to be one of the
common causes of problems for infants who are responsive to cranial
osteopathy. However, a comparison of the explanations offered to
Sarah and to Eileen illustrates a factor which is of concern. Sarah

remembered her difficulty in selecting a practitioner and then making an appointment.

> 6.6: Richard and Sarah – a normal delivery caused the problem
>
> Richard: Well, they do give priority to babies, or cancellations. Because, obviously, a baby who's crying and the earlier they're seen the better. It affects the results that they get. Whilst they don't claim to be able to cure anything, certainly osteopathy has a good success rate.
>
> Sarah: Well, what he actually says is that whatever it is that is wrong in the stomach goes up into the head, and if there's pressure on the brain that causes the problem. If they've had a normal delivery and therefore it's causing pressure on the brain, which is something that links the stomach and the brain. So, if you release the pressure in the brain it relieves the pain in the stomach.
>
> Richard: I wasn't aware it was so common. He actually says that he wishes he could have access to every baby delivery room so he could do it straight away and sort these bones out in the head.

This was an explicit assertion that normal vaginal delivery causes the problem of excessive crying because of pressure on the baby's skull during passage through the birth canal. Eileen received a rather different rationale.

> 6.7: Eileen – Birth by Caesarian section caused the problem
>
> She was two months old when we took her to the osteopath, wasn't she? [Nod from Phil to confirm.] He basically said to us, 'How was she born?' So we told him it was a section, and he said she wasn't quite ready to come out and it's, like, everything happens in a complete rush. You're opened up and she pops out into the air. That's it. Her first arrival into the world. It wasn't, like,

introduce the world through a normal delivery. He said it
was something to do with that.

In this case it was alleged that failure to undergo a normal delivery, coupled with the psychological trauma to the baby of a sudden transition from uterus to delivery room, had caused the crying. Sarah was also told that:

Sometimes the bone structure in the head is as it is anyway,
and it causes pressure, but if there's a rapid delivery or a long
delivery, or sometimes just the way the baby's been laid...

The list of circumstances which allegedly indicate referral for cranial osteopathy, from what participants were told or understood would appear to include:

- Normal delivery
- Forceps delivery
- Caesarean section
- Rapid delivery
- Long delivery
- Natural skull bone structure
- Position in utero such as to crush the skull bones.

All of these and more besides are listed as problems that cranial osteopathy can help with.[3]

Clearly, this leaves little to chance, with few babies escaping all of these factors. (Presumably the inclusion of normal delivery and Caesarean section limits the scope for manoeuvre somewhat.) The list of infantile and childhood conditions that are susceptible to cranial osteopathy includes...

...glue ear, migraine, dizziness, the effects of difficult or
prolonged deliveries in babies and children, as well as
orthopaedic and spinal conditions for which other osteopathic techniques would be inappropriate.[4]

Additionally, the Osteopathic Centre for Children suggests that

Paediatric osteopathy can be used to treat children with a
wide range of conditions, from relatively minor ailments
through to asthma, epilepsy, contagious diseases and
cerebral palsy.[5]

The Osteopathic Home Page suggests that osteopathy can be used to treat...

> ...colic, nursing problems, spitting up, constipation, allergies, asthma, colds, scoliosis, increased tendency to become ill/recurrent illnesses, strains, sprains, learning disabilities, failure to thrive, cerebral palsy, strabismus, torticollis, postural problems, etc.[6]

A list previously featured on the GOsC website was followed by the simple suggestion that vaccination can be responsible for many of the problems addressed by cranial osteopathy.[7] The scientific basis for the whole practice of cranial osteopathy is as yet seriously lacking, although the profession has admirable aims. Claims such as those made above to knowledge of causation of excessive crying, and irresponsible comments about side effects of vaccination do damage to osteopathy's cause. The promise of such a panacea is a strong attractor for families so desperate for a cure. Unfortunately, for the families concerned, their encounter with osteopathy left them with more disappointment after yet another failure in the search for a cure, moderately worse off financially, and sometimes with increased feelings of guilt. As Eileen mused, 'Perhaps if I hadn't needed a section...'

Expecting a cure: encounters with doctors

When a baby is presented by parents complaining about excessive crying careful assessment is clearly required. Sometimes the reason for the crying may be readily apparent and easily remedied. Obviously inappropriate parenting techniques or strategies are commonly addressed by health visitors, usually with a satisfactory outcome. Similarly, common childhood ailments are frequently diagnosed by GPs and for some of these effective remedies are to be had or the parents can be reassured of a self-limiting minor illness which will resolve quickly and with only supportive therapy.

Numerous suggestions have been made to guide the GP's investigation of a case of excessive infantile crying (eg Reust and Blake 2000). The physician's task should not be underestimated, however. In a case of excessive crying the parents are likely to be anxious and exhausted. The baby will usually present with common symptoms (not feeding well, crying 'all the time', not sleeping well, irritable) which may be symptomatic of a great many illnesses and problems. The list of differential diagnoses can be very long. If, after examining a thoroughly unhappy baby and untangling a convoluted history from the parents the doctor concludes that the baby has 'colic' (or, perhaps, that this is one of those cases in which there is no pathological cause to be found and the crying will just resolve in time) then they are faced with a number of treatment choices, each with inconclusive evidence of efficacy. It will be seen that the lack of a firm diagnosis and associated specific treatment can be very difficult for parents to accept, and this may lead to negative estimations of the medical effort to help. Subsequent consultations are often equally lacking in the desired outcome for parents (whatever the reality of what can be offered), and, presumably, equally frustrating for the GP.

Moreover, lurking in the background for the doctor is the constant possibility that, although rare, a baby with such vague symptoms who otherwise appears well may be developing something much more sinister. Ruiz-Contreras et al (1999), for example, report the cases of two infants who were diagnosed as suffering from colic but were found up to 10 hours later to have serious sepsis which could have become life-threatening. This is not an indictment on the competence of the physician, but an indication of the difficulties involved when trying to distinguish between the numerous cases in which the baby may be placed at risk through hospitalisation and those (far more rare) in which serious illness may be about to declare itself. Such diagnostic matters must remain the concern of texts dedicated to the subject, but it is important for other practitioners to be aware of the issues in their own dealings with the parents.

Parental dissatisfaction with the medical profession has been found in a number of studies (for example, Ley 1988, Bradford 1997) and this dissatisfaction was a recurrent feature of the interviews in this study, too. A small part of an interview with Melanie and Mike raised many of the issues which need to be considered. Mike offered insights into their numerous visits to the surgery.

6.8: Mike – Being fobbed off

A lot of the time they all said the same thing. It's just like a fob-off isn't it? To me, that's an easy way out for them. You know what I mean? They can't be bothered finding out properly, or they just don't know and they won't admit it. Now I could live with it if they said, 'We haven't a clue why your baby's crying like this. Some just do this and you have to wait until it goes away.' Then I could live with it. Fine. There's nothing we can do to stop it. What can we do to make it easier? Is there any medication to

> make her sleep more or something? And how long will it
> go on for? When will it stop? You see, they don't tell you
> that. I don't think that they're interested, really. They don't
> believe what you say. They think you're exaggerating.

Several of the parents felt that they had been fobbed off. They perceived that doctors had little inclination to take the problem seriously, and were not motivated to pursue the cause of the crying further. They failed to meet the parents' important need for information, reassurance, and restoration of self-confidence. A long list of alleged failings can appear to the uncritical to be self-evident and to constitute proof of the allegations. While the medical profession must undoubtedly contain within its ranks practitioners whose attitude, knowledge or skills fall below the accepted minimum standard, it is to be hoped that these remain the exception rather than the rule. The catalogue of dissatisfaction was made up of several elements.

Parents often wished for more information to be forthcoming from medical practitioners. This was expressed in a variety of ways, but Phil was very clear.

6.9: Phil – needing more information

> I think what I would have liked from the GP is a little more
> explanation to describe the symptoms of the condition. If
> they said, 'She will scream the house down at five o'clock
> in the morning, and she will look like someone is sticking
> a hot iron into her back, but don't worry about it, it's just
> colic.' But nobody said that. It was just, like, 'Oh yes, they
> cry a lot.' Well, you need to be told more than that. I
> wouldn't say that the medical profession have been sup-
> portive in any way. I reckon it's because they don't know.
> They just fob you off. The doctor was a waste of time.

These were harsh words but they expressed not only the need for information but also the anxiety associated with the frightening symptoms displayed by their baby. The information was sought to eliminate this lack of understanding in the hope of learning which symptoms were significant and which could be accepted or ignored. Phil and Eileen were not alone in their concern. Some parents felt ignorant and unsure. 'For me it's that helplessness and that lack of knowing what's OK and what's not,' explained Alan. 'Is it normal for him to cry so much? Can it do any harm? How will we know when there's a good sign? And worse than that, how do we know that he's getting worse and we should be taking him down to the doctor's?' Susan and her mother shared this last concern in particular. They both worried frequently about decisions regarding when to consult the GP; unwilling to seek a consultation needlessly yet anxious not to fail the baby should he be in real need. Helen's GP had examined Michael thoroughly but, finding no pathology, she advised Helen to give Michael paracetamol. Helen wanted to know the reason for this.

6.10: Helen – I need to know what's wrong

She examined him and said she couldn't hear anything for him screaming. She couldn't listen to his heart or his breathing noises because he was just too loud. So she said to take him home and give him paracetamol. So I asked what was wrong with him. I mean, why give paracetamol if there was nothing wrong with him? I wasn't happy with just giving him paracetamol without knowing why. It says it on the bottle, doesn't it? Not to give it before three months. Now there's a reason for that, presumably? But this doctor was saying, 'We don't know what's wrong with him, but give him Calpol.' I needed to know what was wrong with him.

In this case Helen appeared to be cautious, requiring a rationale before administering apparently contraindicated medication. Others simply saw no therapeutic value in the medication prescribed for their baby. A minority, like Peter, took more personal offence from encounters with doctors, feeling that they were not being taken seriously.

6.11 Peter – I want a better response from you. Believe me.

We still feel that they didn't believe us. That was the annoying part. You know? I felt like, 'I'm an adult here. I'm not a 10-year-old kid. I'm an adult. I'm having to put up with this all the time and I want some better response from you.' But we just got this response: 'What are you worried about? He's OK.' They've got to tell you more. You need the information to be able to put up with this.

The height of indignation was reached by Joyce when she visited her GP with Matthew whose crying had grown progressively more intense. 'I took him to the doctor and he said it was most probably because it was a full moon!' Another pointed example of a perceived patronising approach was provided by Julie, who was qualified and experienced in child care, and was seeking help with her second child.

6.12: Julie – Don't patronise me!

> Well, my GP told me that it was my fault that she was screaming. She said, 'If you lay her across your legs, pat her back a couple of times, it'll get rid of all that wind out of her tummy.' And I said, 'What! How can you say this is all my fault? I'm bringing all her wind up. I'm doing all I can.' 'Well, you're obviously not getting all her wind up, then, are you?' I was absolutely livid... I lost all confidence in the GP... She was a waste of time. In fact, she probably made me worse, because I came away from there in tears.

The validity of this as an exact recollection of the meeting, and its representative status with regard to consultations with GPs could, of course be contested. However, the key factor is the outcome of a dissatisfied client who has found disappointment in her quest for information, support and practical assistance. This general concern with information was heightened in the expectation that every possible appropriate test or investigation would be undertaken. Superficial physical examination would not suffice.

It was interesting to find that the demand for testing and information as a result was not necessarily linked to expectations of a positive outcome or of consequent treatment options. Sarah and Richard were among those who sought investigations more in the hope of prognostic information than of a cure. Richard seemed fairly resigned to finding no cure, but he felt a need to know what to expect.

6.13: Do tests - try harder to find out

> It would help to know more. At least if they do the test and say there's nothing significantly wrong, that he was fine, but might continue for the next four or five months that would be OK. And there again, if they could say that it is only a minor thing that sometimes happens then that would certainly help. It would put your mind at rest.
>
> (Richard)

> I got sick of being told, 'It's just one of those things.' That was no use at all. I wanted them to do something to find out more, even if it was only so that... I'd much rather be

> told that there is an end in sight: that it's not going to go
> on for ever. But 'Just one of those things!' If they were try-
> ing they wouldn't come out with tosh like 'It's just one of
> those things.' That's just a cop-out.   (Helen)

At this point it is important to remember the guilt that parents often feel because of their inability to settle the baby and their ever-present concern that they should be doing more to seek a cause and a cure. Richard wanted medical investigation to demonstrate that nothing had been missed and that the crying was a harmless aberration which was self-limiting and would terminate at a given point. This was the case for Helen, too.

The overall evaluation by participants of the response from doctors was not favourable. Discounting the occasional incidence of inappropriate attitude and deliberate obtuseness, however, the GPs and paediatricians appeared mostly to have fulfilled their basic function of diagnosis and prescription as far as circumstances allowed. Their diagnoses may not have been what was hoped for, and the success of their prescriptions was drastically limited. Yet this was all, perhaps, inevitable. As explained earlier, parents sought a clear diagnosis to explain the crying and a prescription bearing a guarantee of success. Neither was a real possibility. Even a diagnosis of 'colic' represents only a formal (and variable) description of the symptoms. Further investigation would not improve the specificity of the diagnosis; a cure was not to be had; and the prognosis had to remain a mystery.

Perhaps improvements could be made in the manner of presenting the details to parents, and more effort made to demonstrate sincere interest during consultations. Certainly, Bradford (1997, 159) found similar reactions to those detailed above in his study of parents of chronically ill children.

> I drew attention to the way the medical system's manage-
> ment of the emotional aspects of the child and family's care
> was a significant source of dissatisfaction. It seemed that
> the organisation of services often meant that parents failed
> to have their emotional needs met, thereby adding further
> barriers to successful coping. Underlying this was a failure
> in communication, whereby parents frequently failed to ask
> the questions they wanted, and clinicians and others failed
> to meet their needs for information, discussion and emo-
> tional support. It seems that parents commonly complained
> that they were not told enough and that the way in which
> they were given information was unsatisfactory too.

While this correlates well with the findings from this study, dissatis-faction would probably persist even if efforts were made to address the specific items detailed in Bradford's study and in this one. The enforced brevity of medical consultation events; their location remote from the site of the problem; and their isolated nature in the context of the wider difficulties for the family may often condemn the doctor's efforts to fail-ure in the eyes of the parents.

Responding with support: the role of the health visitor

The factors that led to the common, and perhaps almost inevitable, phenomenon of parental disappointment with medical intervention were equally forceful in the development of perceptions of the role of the health visitor, whose intervention was almost universally viewed in a positive light by participants. Four elements in particular represented the needs that were apparently able to be met by health visitors. The parents, while recognising that only a fellow sufferer could truly under-stand the experience, wanted professionals (or anyone else) to listen and at least to try to understand. The therapeutic value of taking the time to talk was an integral part of this. The second need was simply to be believed. The effect of parents' perception that doctors did not believe them is laid out above. Taking these two elements further, par-ents especially valued any time when a relative or health professional (in practice always a health visitor in this study) spent time with them on a prolonged or regular basis. The need was for someone in a sup-portive capacity to be with, or stay with, the participant and to share the anguish and stress provoked by the crying. Finally, the parents sought reassurance on three specific issues: that they were not to blame for the crying; that there was no intervention that they had missed; and that the crying would stop eventually.

The need for support and how this may be met were clear enough, then, and such need was not being met through the services of doctors or osteopaths. Midwives, whose role in this area is normally limited anyway to the first month after the baby's birth, played little part in the families' lives. There were only three incidences of midwives being mentioned in the whole of the interview transcript material. These indicated only that midwives had played no part in addressing the cry-ing, or that they had not taken an active interest in the issue (attending instead to physical, clinical matters). The reasons for this were beyond the bounds of this study, and no speculation is made here about the benefits, failings, or potential for therapeutic intervention from mid-wives. There was one health professional, however, whose intervention was found to be at least potentially beneficial and whose efforts were appreciated by the families. This was the health visitor.

> 6.14: Joanne – I'd not waste my time. I'd go straight to the health visitor
>
> I think the health visitor is 10 times more important than the doctor. If it's something medical like a sty or something, then I'd go straight to the doctor. But if I was worried otherwise I'd not waste my time: I'd go straight to the health visitor.

The explanation for Joanne's attitude can be found by considering each of the four main needs for support and assessing the health visitor's contribution to these. Since this aspect of the emerging theory became clearer in the latter half of the study, contributions from those interviews (Helen, Julie and Elaine, particularly) offer the clearest expressions to illustrate the matters at hand and may be seen to predominate.

The need for people to listen and to try to understand

> 6.15: People don't even try to understand
>
> They don't know how it is. It's hard. Unless you're a mother who's had the same, no-one can understand what you've been through. You'll never know how awful it can be. But you could try. I wanted someone to see what was going on and then recognise how awful it was for me.
>
> (Julie)
>
> You see, I don't think you could ever really understand what it's like until you've had one yourself, but it seemed to me that people weren't even trying to understand. Except for the health visitor.   (Helen)

The inability to understand without first-hand experience need not prevent a health professional intervening effectively, then. The key lay in attempting to understand and being seen to do so. Several participants remarked on the benefit of talking about the problem, either within the family or to a professional. However, this indicated a facility for the parent to talk, with the implicit requirement that the professional would listen. The limitation of this intervention in isolation, even by someone who had suffered the same plight, was also highlighted by Helen, who said:

> I spoke to Cry-sis. Although it was good to talk to someone
> who knew what I was talking about, sort of mutual aid or
> something, I really wanted her to say, 'Do this, or do that
> and it will be all right.' I was still searching for a solution.

Talking, listening, and trying to understand may be more important as a means to gain trust and provide a foundation for more effective intervention. It should, perhaps, be considered one of a raft of mutually supportive or integral strategies.

6.16: Just needing someone to listen

> Oh, my health visitor was brilliant. I mean, as far as they
> can do. They can only offer to listen to you, but that made
> such a change. She would listen all day if I carried on.
>
> (Joyce)

> I've gone to her and said, 'I just need to talk,' and they lis-
> ten to you. I can ring them up at any time, in work time,
> obviously, but she'll listen to me or she'll come and visit
> me. You know: just to listen. So I've been really fortunate,
> then.   (Janet)

Field (1994), in a survey to compare mothers' and nurses' reliance on specific symptoms to diagnose colic in the baby, found that the two groups differed substantially on which symptoms were most important. The implication of this might be that nurses would fail to address or recognise the significance of mother's reported concerns. However, the participants in this study reported quite the opposite. Joyce was obviously impressed with her health visitor's attempt to meet this need to listen and to try to understand. She valued the opportunity to speak at length with a professional about her difficulties; to be able to include all the more minor issues which together contributed a significant amount to the problem. Similar appreciation was expressed by Janet.

6.17: Just try to understand

> People tried to be supportive. The health visitor and the
> breast-feeding counsellor, who was also a health visitor,
> certainly tried to be supportive, although they didn't

know what else to suggest. Perhaps if we had all realised then that they were helping just by taking notice. I don't think I even realised it myself until now.   (Elaine)

I really felt like she wanted to know and wanted to understand. Now, that was unusual. I felt like I could talk to her and have him screaming in the background and it was OK… People weren't even trying to understand. Except for the health visitor.   (Helen)

Elaine recognised the apparent limitations of what could physically be achieved but, nevertheless, acknowledged the contribution made by people simply trying to understand and to help. Helen's health visitor also demonstrated the commitment to understanding that was sought. So when the health visitor made the effort to engage meaningfully with the family and its problems this was noticed and appreciated. Trying to understand was sufficient: it demonstrated commitment and sincerity, and it opened the way for further investment by the health visitor.

The need to be believed

6.18: Julie – I'm not exaggerating!

I just wanted the health visitor to know I was having a bad time: that the screaming was as bad as it was. Trying to get that across to her, well to anybody, that's the hardest thing… That was a lot of it, you see, I just felt that people thought I was making it up or putting it on. People thought I was exaggerating it.

Perceiving that people did not believe the intensity of the problem was a significant aspect of the difficulty of coping with excessive crying, and this was particularly pronounced with regard to professionals. Most participants expressed the need to be believed, and several commented that their health visitor appeared to satisfy this need. Having offered a lengthy description of unsatisfactory encounters with doctors, Roisin considered the contribution made by other professionals.

6.19: Roisin – When I tell her, she believes me

The health visitor [named health visitor]. She's the only one. She really believed us when we said what it was like…

She will sit and listen to me and she wants to know, and
when I tell her, she believes me. She just sits there and says,
'Did you have a bad night? How's he been?' And I tell her
and you can see that she doesn't think I'm exaggerating.
She's bloody good.

Echoes of this could be heard in the words of Sarah and Richard who
each considered whether there was any point in the health visitor call-
ing if there was nothing that could be done to stop the crying. 'Oh, yes,'
Sarah asserted. 'Just having somebody coming to listen and to answer
questions makes a difference. More than that, it's having somebody tell
you they believe you.' 'Yes,' agreed Richard. 'Just to know somebody's
on your side. You feel like there's two of you then against the world. So
it's not just me on my own.'

Julie, too, found relief when her health visitor stated explicitly that
she accepted what she was being told about the crying. Nicola had
played true to form, and when the health visitor called, in Julie's words,
she 'tuned up'. The health visitor said, 'Oh, yes. I can see that you've
got a real problem there. This must be really stressful.' From there it was
possible to consider a wide range of issues about the family's health and
the issue of the crying. The visit helped Julie to recognise some of the
good things that were still happening in her life, and that despite the
crying, Nicola was developing well, as was her sister, Lucy. These comments and episodes do something to demonstrate the importance for
parents of being believed and feeling that a professional was supportive
of them and was 'on their side'.

The need for someone to visit and 'be there'

The final need that was commonly expressed was for someone to be
with the parent, to spend time in their company offering moral support
and breaking the isolation reinforced by living with the crying day
after day.

6.20: Elaine – Someone to take the time and be there for
you, at home

You feel helpless. So with that and the guilt you can end up
feeling fairly bad about the whole thing. So if other people
don't or perhaps won't understand that makes it all the
harder to cope. Maybe that's why it's still good for people
to come: the health visitor and the breast-feeding counsellor. Just so someone understands or at least tries to.

> Someone who will not judge you, but will sympathise and
> support you and help you through it. If they just take the
> time and be there for you, at home, and give you the time
> that you need. I don't even know what they would do. But
> it still seems important for them to come and be there.

For some the need to have someone call at the house to assist with the coping process was rather vague. Elaine appeared to be clarifying the issues for herself as she spoke. Julie was a little clearer about her need. 'It's all right her coming once when I'm having a bad time, but why can't they come more often and just check that everything's all right?' She knew, in fact, that the main reason was a lack of resources, but she was simply expressing her need. 'I know she's got other people to see, but when you're really struggling you don't want to know that, do you?' She saw great benefit in the visit that she received from her health visitor, but knew that she could gain even more from more frequent and more prolonged contact.

6.21: Helen – Showing commitment and time

> Well, the health visitor helped in another way. She would
> just come and hang around the house with me for an hour
> or two. This was even after we'd gone through all the
> things that you can do and nothing had worked. She used
> to come at least twice a week at one point... It was a strat-
> egy that she used because I did cope and get through.

The means by which the health visitor could help was more obvious to Helen. Everything had been tried and had failed, yet it helped just for the health visitor to be there, sharing the experience for a while and showing commitment in time and emotional effort.

Muriel and Diane, Malachy's grandmother and aunt respectively, recognised their role in supporting his mother in this manner. Apart from the physical assistance with housework and taking turns at holding the baby, they realised that simply being in the house with Susan was therapeutic for her. As the immediate family is usually the main source of support it takes little analysis to see that family members are more likely than anyone else to be able to meet all four requirements laid out here: to understand how life is for the parents; to spend time talking and listening; to believe the parents' account of their lives; and to be with them for support and practical assistance.

6.22: Julie – Help me to cope, here, with the kids

My mum would think that she would take the kids out of
the way and that would help, but that wasn't what I
wanted. I wanted to be with the kids myself. I wanted her
to stay with me and spend some time with me and help
me. It was always easier if my friend came. I just wanted
someone to be with me and help me. That's what I wanted more than anything.

This was not necessarily straightforward, though, and even the best-
intentioned could misinterpret their relative's need. Julie desperately
wanted to cope better with her baby – not to have the problem
removed from her. Indeed, giving the baby up to someone else who
might cope better was particularly difficult to contemplate. Julie's
mother's misunderstanding of her daughter's needs reduced the efficacy
of her desire to help and had already led to a rift between them.

6.23: Peter – You felt like she was never far away

She [the health visitor] used to come round here. We used
to bump into her all the time. She'd always know who
you were, even me, so you always felt good with her.
Relaxed. She always knew about us. She always remembered. You'd see her on the estate, going to someone
else's house or whatever. You felt like she was never far
away, somehow.

It was not simply time spent in the house that promoted a feeling of
having someone with a professional background involved in the problem and focused on the family. Peter spoke of the health visitor who
had helped the family to cope with the crying of two of the three children. This, in its own way, is an eloquent description of the family
visitor: the core of the role of the health visitor, serving a local
community and providing a reassuring presence for all.

The need for specific reassurance

In many cases parents perceived themselves to be helpless to change
their wretched situation; they often felt guilt (or were caused to do so
by others) for their assumed part in the problem; they discovered an
unwillingness on the part of those who could help to believe their

allegations or to take them seriously; and they had a desperate need for a reliable, sensitive confidant who, while unable to improve everything in their life, could make a positive difference.

The need to be believed has been dealt with above. Feelings of guilt were intimately linked to this. Melanie recognised her need for help particularly because of her inexperience in child care.

> 6.24: Melanie – Keep telling me that it's not my fault

> I think probably it was reassurance. Yes. That was it: reassurance. Because I was a first-time mother I needed things explaining and I always thought it was just me. But my health visitor kept telling me it wasn't my fault. That was good. I needed that.

The guilt discussed previously clearly could be negated by someone with the knowledge to state with authority that it was not the parents' fault. The guilt could relate to fear that some potential cure or treatment had been missed or ignored by the parent, or that the parent was actively causing the problem because of poor child care skills. As a young first-time mother, coping for part of the time alone, Melanie was susceptible to the latter anxiety.

Others, such as Claire, who was caring for her second child, felt more concern about having omitted to try every possible treatment. The need to be reassured that 'it's not your fault' could stem from more than one source, but the message did not vary.

> 6.25: Claire – Tell me that I've not missed anything

> Reassurance was certainly needed sometimes. Even though I felt sure that I'd done everything there was to do, and tried everything there was to try, I couldn't help feeling like there had to be something else... I had to carry on looking for an answer. Maybe if someone had told me that there wasn't an answer I could have accepted it. I don't know whether health visitors would have time to visit just to give reassurance like that, but perhaps that would help. You know: it can make a big difference that there is somebody there to tell you that there isn't anything wrong with them, that you've not missed anything, and there isn't anything else to be done.

What remained was the need to be reassured that the crying would stop eventually. Parents experienced difficulty in seeing ahead to a time when the crying would no longer be a problem. When the possibility of supportive intervention was discussed more concrete (and, perhaps, positive) wishes were expressed. Speaking of her desire for the health visitor or breast-feeding counsellor to attend, be supportive and sympathise, Elaine concluded, 'Perhaps you even need reminding that it will come right some time. If there was someone who could do that they'd be an angel, wouldn't they?' Julie had suggested that more frequent visits by the health visitor would be effective. 'Well, she could have told me all that time ago that it wasn't my fault: that I wasn't doing anything wrong. Maybe she could have rammed it home that it will stop eventually.' Helen also wanted – and received – this support.

> 6.26: Helen – psychological boost
>
> Yes. She'd made all the suggestions she could. She never said he was abnormal. She said, 'There are some babies who do this. Take heart: he'll grow out of it.' When she came we would go for a walk with the pram and she would come with us. He would be screaming but it didn't seem to put her off. That helped. That boosted me. Psychologically that boosted me. Just when I was feeling most isolated she would come and listen and be shouted at.

When doctors stated to parents that there was nothing to be done about the crying; that it would stop sometime; and that they would just have to cope, their attitude was questioned and their contribution dismissed. Here was a health visitor giving the same message but being received warmly and found to be a positive, therapeutic force. The difference must be seen to lie in the isolation of the doctor's pronouncement from the other three elements of parents' needs: the time and effort spent listening and trying to understand, the explicit assertion of believing the parent, and the extended presence at the site of the event are vital components, too.

Notes

1. http://www.cry-sis.com/cryingbaby.html (accessed 07.03.04)
2. http://www.osteopathy.org.uk 'Your questions answered FAQs' 2003
3. http://www.osteopathy.org.uk. A link from the GOsC pages to 'The Osteopathic Home Page' leads to http://www.osteohome.com/mainPages/children.html. This page details a wide range of paediatric medical conditions susceptible to osteopathy (including colic).

4. http://www.osteopathy.org.uk/ois/factsheets/e.shtml (Accessed 29.12.03)
5. http://www.occ.uk.com/info/info.html (Accessed 29.12.03)
6. http://www.osteohome.com/MainPages/children.html (Accessed 29.12.03)
7. Cranial osteopathy for babies, infants and children. http://www.users.dircon.co.uk (Accessed in 1999)

Chapter 7
Concluding remarks

The scope of these conclusions

It is clear from Chapter 2 that confusion reigns over the precise definition of what constitutes excessive crying. In this book 'colic' as a term has been found to be lacking in view of its variable, dissonant definitions, its uncertain distinction from excessive crying, and the evidence from parents that its status is more an aspect or phase of excessive crying than a discrete diagnosis or problem. This is not to deny, however, that the terms excessive crying and colic will continue to be used interchangeably by both lay and professional individuals regardless. For reasons argued in Chapter 2 the perspective has been adopted that excessive crying as a problem is best defined by those who report it. This strategy, while perhaps adding nothing to epidemiological efforts, at least offers the greatest chance of effective intervention by professionals.

The study on which much of the conclusions are based dealt with families who had tried all the common interventions aimed at resolving the crying and often less common, more radical suggestions, too. This text addresses living and coping with excessive crying which resists all of these efforts. As was repeatedly asserted by participants: nothing worked. Perhaps the majority of those who experience problems with more infantile crying than they expected find relief in standard interventions, and these comments refer only to those who fail at this point.

Disrupted lives

The lives of the families were characterised by pervasive disruption. Almost every aspect of life, both physical and psychological, was affected. Relationships between parents grew strained, siblings suffered, guilt accumulated, and daily life became a chaotic rush: running just to keep up. A number of factors combined to promote social isolation, a gradual introversion with the crying becoming the focus of life. The absence of any period of relief from the daily grind of coping with the crying and its associated effects eventually caused exhaustion and loss of control. The most significant fear for parents from this was the danger of non-accidental injury to the baby. Such fears, exhaustion, and the occurrence of intermittent periods of especially heightened tension, led to a pattern of approaching and withdrawing from a point of total loss of control: living on the edge. Acknowledgement of this spasmodic proximity to a regretful incident further fed the guilt, stress and desperation of parents.

This disruption was too severe and prolonged simply to be tolerated, so active efforts had to be made to secure an improvement. Indeed, a significant part of the guilt experienced by parents arose from interpreting inability to correct the progressive slide into chaos as inadequate parenting and culpable ignorance. Of course, popular literature and some professional approaches reinforced this perception. Two avenues of action were open to parents, but for several reasons one of these was far more attractive than the other. Cultural and societal expectations, and the focus of the National Health Service, led firstly (and repeatedly) to a search for a diagnosis.

Search for a diagnosis

As more consultations were attended and the desired result was not attained, the sense of disappointment and despondency grew. Options were seen to be used up and a final stalemate foreseen. When it became clear that traditional medicine had no solution, or even a convincing explanation for the crying, parents would often turn to alternative therapies. There is nothing unique to excessive crying in this: the use of alternative and complementary therapies as a last resort is a feature of many illnesses for which no common cure exists. Unfortunately for the parents in this study, however, no relief was to be found in this part of their quest for a cure either. So the search for a diagnosis and consequent cure was doomed to failure, but the alternative seemed so unbearable that attempts to find a cause could not be abandoned. Life and morale spiralled through a repetitive sequence of hope, active search and disappointment. There were varying periods of resigned acceptance that a cure would not be found and life settled down (comparatively) to a steady, resigned plod. Little stimulation was needed, however, for the peace to be shattered and the pursuit of ever-more dubious causes or unlikely strategies to be resumed. The revolutions of hope, active search and disappointment may be seen as a recurrent tumble towards, and retreat from, an abyss representing loss of control and an untoward incident, perhaps including non-accidental injury. This, naturally, provoked major concern and prolonged anxiety for parents.

For some this cycle endured until the problem eventually ran its course, the baby grew older, and the crying gradually subsided. This could take as long as a year, and behavioural problems could persist for a further year or more. For others, a second strategic approach could be employed: that of support through the problem, enhancing coping until the crying went away of its own accord.

The response from professionals

Apart from each other, for most parents the greatest source of support in coping, both practical and psychological, was the immediate family, notably grandparents. Once the parents' specific needs for support were identified it was easy to see why this should be so, but also to recognise the enormous potential and demand for professional intervention. Four specific needs required attention.

1. The need for people to listen and to try to understand
2. The need to be believed
3. The need for someone to visit and to 'be there'.
4. The need for reassurance that the parents were not to blame and that the crying would stop eventually.

The constraints of medical practice in both time and location militated against an effective role with regard to the first three of these. Furthermore, although well qualified to address the last need, prognosis being a vital and legitimate component of medical practice, doctors would normally fail in this, too. The GP's honest assessment that no cure was available but that the crying would stop eventually was usually interpreted as lack of interest and avoidance of effort. While general expectations of a diagnosis and treatment for all illnesses may have contributed to this, the major cause was the lack of investment in the first three needs.

Demonstration of belief in the parents' story was a vital element of establishing rapport and gaining trust. Explicit verbal confirmation of belief was essential, but more active, persistent reinforcement was necessary. A visible commitment to trying to understand the parents' difficulties had to be made: a time-consuming business requiring skills of active listening and demonstration of empathy. There is sufficient evidence that those who complain to professionals that their baby cries excessively do, indeed, have a baby who cries more often and for longer than most. Belief in this, and in the pervasive effects that the crying exerts on the whole family, was the basic requirement for a professional to be accepted and trusted to proceed further into the depths of the parents' world.

Having established a relationship with parents the next issue to be addressed was the perception of guilt, that the crying was attributable to acts or omissions on the parents' part. Most parents needed to be told repeatedly, convincingly, and with sincerity that they were not to blame. Although examples were found of parents being explicitly accused of poor parenting practice, more often the feelings of guilt resulted from self-recrimination or perhaps from perceptions of external criticism. It seems that even though parents may have known that they had acted in a proper and responsible manner, exhausting every means of helping the baby, they could not rid themselves of thoughts of having failed. Such self-doubt could not easily be countered. It demanded repeated confirmation from someone with the authority of professional knowledge and who had already established a commitment to the family that no potential solutions had been missed. There needed to be an explicit assertion that the crying was not the fault of the parents, and skill was needed in persuading them to accept this. Hearing such reassuring messages and being convinced was clearly therapeutic, and the therapy was needed in repeated doses, sometimes on a frequent basis. Self-recrimination might be expected to peak when parents felt 'close to the edge' and to wane as life returned to a more settled routine, but it was always present, persisting long after the crying had abated. Health professionals working with such families months after the episode of excessive crying might expect to find residual effects and feelings of guilt.

Both of these issues responded better to intervention which was prolonged and situated in the home. A major part of the reason for the perceived failing of medicine was its location distant from the scene of the problem and the unavoidable brevity of consultations. Parents felt a need for someone to address their problems in the home, taking time to experience a greater breadth of the difficulties being faced, and giving further evidence of a commitment to see the problem through to the end. While acknowledging the current impossibility of their demands, parents expressed in unambiguous terms their need for visits to occur perhaps three times per week, or even daily, and to last for two or three hours each time. Periods of feeling close to the edge provoked greater need for this prolonged professional presence, but this was less

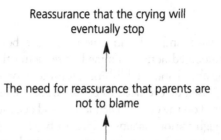

Reassurance that the crying will
eventually stop

The need for reassurance that parents are
not to blame

The need for people to believe and to try to understand

The need for someone to 'be there' frequently and for prolonged periods

Figure 7.1: The relationship of needs for support.

pronounced during less traumatic periods. The linkage between this requirement of prolonged domiciliary contact and those of being believed and reassured about lack of guilt was an intimate one. Each necessitated a major allocation of time and emotional effort. 'Being there' was a way of confirming commitment to the family; it increased the chances of coming to understand the situation better; and it enhanced the credibility of reassuring assertions.

The final need was for the message to be driven home that the crying would stop in time. Although logically this may seem superfluous, since babies will obviously eventually grow older and stop crying, there was a specific need. In the chaos and unceasing grind of coping on a daily basis with excessive crying it could be remarkably difficult to accept or draw comfort from the inevitability of an ultimate resolution. Projecting forward to a time when life would be normal and more enjoyable required assurance firstly that the crying would, indeed, stop within a foreseeable period, and, secondly, that no residual effects should be expected. There would be no developmental, psychological or physical impairment or sequelae. This assurance could not be provided adequately in a brief consultation however knowledgeable and authoritative the professional might be. Successful intervention in this key area demanded attention first to the previous three aspects of need.

A pyramidal structure may be used to represent the relationship of these needs (see Figure 7.1) in which resolution of each need is reliant upon a satisfactory outcome of those below.

Coping

Coping was found to be an issue relating to both problem-focused and emotion-focused activities aimed at reducing the threat to family life. Planning ahead and establishing a routine in order to regain control was counterpoised by the need to break out of the enforced boundaries of a life focused on the crying. Distraction and occasional relief from the crying through various means helped to bolster coping, and varying risks could be seen as being temporarily acceptable in order to secure such a break. Parents looked primarily to each other for practical and psychological support, and sharing the load between them was a vital part of their survival tactics. They experienced alternating periods of peaks and troughs of coping, with few predictable factors to account for the switch from one to the other. However, the recognition of minor victories and up-lifts of mood for whatever reason could often stimulate an improvement. There were periods of relative stability which were characterised by resignation to the effects of the crying and re-adjustment of expectations. The inevitability of the crying stopping eventually could not be accepted while coping was in a trough and while more immediate demands and fatigue obliterated such optimistic assertions. The repeated disappointments of failures of potential cures added to this and often prevented recognition of the minor or gradual improvements that heralded eventual resolution of the problem.

The role of the health visitor

It will be obvious from the study, and it was explicitly suggested by participants, that there is one prime candidate for the role of professional intervention in the case of intractable excessive crying. This is the health visitor. Health visitors, by the requirements of their professional preparation and practice, already possess the knowledge, skills and motivation to undertake the task. Sufficient time, the necessary resources, and wider recognition of the potential of the health visitor are all sadly lacking, however.

Focus on parents and families

The effects of social isolation and the almost universal reliance on partners as a first (and sometimes only) line of support necessitates an approach which is family-centred and supportive specifically of parents. Addressing the needs of families, particularly those with children under five years, is recognised as being a crucial part of the health visitor's role by Botes (1998). Botes also notes the potential for health visitors to organise, lead, or support community developments which support families. The organised voluntary support in the form of a practically helpful, supportive visitor that was wished for by some respondents could constitute just such a development. The third edition of the Hall Report (Hall 1996) reinforces previous encouragement for health visitors to form partnerships with parents, asserting that supporting parents may be more important (and effective) than attending directly to the children. Within the catalogue of evidence that makes up one report (CPHVA 1998) is the finding that focusing by health visitors on parental morale and emotional needs makes a significant difference to the parents' quality of life. Support for parents in a number of guises and through a variety of media is clearly within the remit and capability of health visitors. Parents in this study, however, expressed that this intervention was effective only when provided at the source of the problems: the family home.

Being there

Cody (1999) highlights the provision of a service within the client's own environment as being a key factor in the therapeutic effect of health visiting, and she regrets the current move away from domiciliary visits in favour of clinic contact. Reducing the number of home visits has been a consistent recommendation of the Hall Report (Hall 1996) with the intention of preserving resources and targeting only the most severe cases. Yet the CPHVA (1998) provides further evidence that the presentation of the service in the family home was a crucial factor in enhancing trust, motivation, co-operation and measurable improvement in families' lives.

Prolonged and frequent contact

Support sometimes needed to be on the basis of frequent and prolonged contact; much more than is currently the norm in health visiting. This more intensive contact was found by Cody (1999) to be a significant issue in establishing a therapeutic approach. There is scope for extension to the existing role, however. Chalmers and Luker (1991) explain that health visitors promote and develop relationships with clients with a view to on-going contact over long periods. These periods may extend over years, so the notion of a professional relationship that is more than transitory is already established. Visiting on a more frequent basis has repeatedly been shown to effect positive changes on the health of individuals and families (CPHVA 1998), one example being that additional visits can increase persistence with breast-feeding and ensure appropriate weaning practices. Both of these were common issues within this study. The value of increasing the frequency of visits is also recognised in government initiatives. The consultation document 'Supporting Families' (Home Office 1998) allowed for extra funding for an enhanced health visitor role which would include more frequent visits to specified groups. One of the examples given was that of parents coping with children with sleep problems. The spirit of this would suggest that excessive crying could attract similar resources. Although designed with a more specific aim, the Sure Start initiative (DfEE 1998), too, recommended the application of resources to provide for additional health visitor sessions in the home, with the specific recommendation of arranging clerical support to release more time for direct health visiting activity. It would appear, then, that the significant increase in time spent with families that is sought by those coping with excessive crying may be possible at least in some areas.

Support through listening, advising and reassuring

The overwhelming effects of excessive crying could make it difficult for parents to recognise the positive, normal aspects of life. Part of the health visitor's role is to identify and demonstrate these to parents. A baby that cries excessively may still be developmentally normal or even advanced. Similarly, the obvious effects of the crying on a sibling could easily mask attainments and progress in other areas. Recognising such positive attributes could help to shift attention away from the crying and provide a more encouraging focus. Skill and sensitivity were required to achieve this, and the centrality and effectiveness of psychological support of clients, employing skills of listening, advising and reassuring is detailed by a number of sources. Kerr et al (1996), for example, provide limited evidence of health visitor intervention in the form of information and advice reducing sleep problems in infants, while the achievements with regard to breast-feeding reported above were brought about in the same manner. Cody (1999) notes the importance of active listening and efforts to support parents to re-establish their self-esteem and regain control in their lives. The facilitation of health-enhancing behaviour, stated by the CPHVA (1997) to be a fundamental principle of practice, is often achieved through this support so it is understandable that Cody (1999) regrets that many health visitors are frustrated that the value of their psychological support is so often not recognised.

Peaks and troughs of coping – living on the edge

The intermittent intensity of stress and coping demanded the identification of the times when families were heading towards the edge and failing to cope effectively. Tyson and Sobschak (1994) argue that professionals need actively to seek out imbalances between the demands on families and their ability to meet these demands. In the United Kingdom this has been pursued as the search for health needs, another fundamental principle of health visiting practice (CPHVA 1997). The individual nature of the response to stress and demands upon the family necessitated a personalised approach such as that adopted in family visits by health visitors. The ability to identify those times when a family was on a downward spiral into a trough of coping was crucial. Although the importance of preventative work in areas such as child protection has been stressed (CPHVA 1998), the timing of intervention is crucial. Botes (1998) discusses the need for health visitors to differentiate between families that, while experiencing difficulty, 'have ways and means to obtain support and may therefore be left to ask for professional help when they need it' and those which are more vulnerable and in need of intervention. She notes that this activity demands the attention of a highly skilled professional. The findings from this study suggest that a further distinction may be made within each family of periods of relative coping and episodes of more distress. In short, health visitors need to recognise whether an individual family is approaching or moving away from the edge. It is at the former point that intervention is indicated. Some parents may recognise this and ask for help; others may not. Of all the health professionals who come into contact with families it is the health visitor who has the most legitimate mode of access in the case of overt difficulties or in the absence of a reported problem.

Interestingly, health visitors themselves may not fully appreciate the efficacy of their supportive presence.

7.1: A health visitor – I go, but there's nothing left to try

I've tried everything for her. You know, all the usual things. The milk, the colic drops, position and everything. None of it has made any difference. I don't know what else I can do. I mean, I go, but there's nothing left to try. Perhaps she'll get something out of talking to you. She wants to talk to you, but she knows you haven't got a magic answer either. But maybe it will do something.

Policy implications

In all, then, the observed and expressed needs of the families encountered in this study would best be attended to by health visitors. They have the knowledge, skills and remit to fulfil the required role. Although effective intervention would be costly in terms of human resources, central government has recognised this need and made some limited provision for pilot schemes. There remains, however, an apparent contradiction in expectations of the future role of the health visitor. The potential development of health visiting (some would say reversion) to public health nursing is currently hotly debated. While health visitors may be well-qualified to make the transition, if this were to mean the relinquishing of home visiting the result for families such as those in this study would be deleterious. However, public health nursing would not, of necessity, remove health visitors from the personal contact in the house that is so much demanded. The decision to retain health visiting as a separate profession to nursing and midwifery (National Health Service Executive 1999) and explicit statements regarding an enhanced role for health visitors in supporting parents and families (Home Office 1998) would appear, however, to recognise the potential for health visitors to make a crucial difference to family health and well-being through their current mode of practice. Certainly, there is also the requirement for health visitors to work within a wider team of professionals providing support for families. The needs of the families discussed here could, theoretically, be equally well met by other professionals provided that the workers were able to satisfy the specific requirements detailed above. Pragmatically, however, health visitors currently form the sole health professional group with the knowledge, skills and access demanded of the role suggested by the results of this study.

There is evidence that an enormous amount of time and effort (and, therefore, financial resource) is expended by general practitioners and health visitors in the current mode of response to excessive crying (St James-Roberts and Halil 1991). Additional costing for multiple attendances at accident and emergency departments should be considered, too. Despite this, the outcome of the current provision is, according to those participating in this study, ineffective and even counterproductive. Although additional home visits by health visitors would incur financial implications it might be considered that existing funding could be better utilised, providing a more effective outcome for families and reducing costs elsewhere.

In conclusion

I was stimulated to undertake this study through the impact exerted upon me by interaction with parents whose lives were characterised by distress, despair and exhaustion brought about by the crying of a baby. Through my discussions with such parents I came to understand something of their disrupted lives, the powerful forces which drive the search for a diagnosis, and their perception of the response from professionals. The result suggests that a specific mode of intervention by the family health visitor could help to bring more positive meaning to life with the crying; to assuage the intense feelings of guilt; to enable parents to project ahead to life without the crying; and to minimise the periods of time spent 'living on the edge' with the concurrent risk of injury to the baby. Such outcomes would make an incalculable difference to the lives of the families affected and may bring substantial professional satisfaction to the health visitors involved in supporting them.

References

Alvarez M, St James-Roberts I (1996) Infant fussing and crying patterns in the first year of life in an urban community in Denmark. Acta Paediatrica 85(4), 463-466.

Baildam E M, Hillier V F, Ward B S, Bannister R P, Bamford F N, Moore W M (1995) Duration and pattern of crying in the first year of life. Developmental Medicine and Child Neurology 37(4), 345-353.

Barr R G (1990) The 'colic' enigma: prolonged episodes of a normal disposition to cry. Infant Mental Health Journal 11, 340-348.

Barr R G (1993) Herbal teas for infantile colic. Journal of Pediatrics 123(4), 669, 670-671.

Barr R G (1998) Crying in the first year of life: good news in the midst of distress. Child: Care, Health and Development 24(5), 425-439.

Barr R G, Elias M F (1988) Nursing interval and maternal responsivity: effect on early infant crying. Pediatrics 81(4), 529-536.

Barr R G, Kramer M S, Boisjoly C, McVey-White I, Pless I B (1988) Parental diary of infant cry and fuss behaviour. Archives of Disease in Childhood 63(4), 380-387.

Barr R G, Kramer M S, Pless I B, Boisjoly C, Leduc D (1989) Feeding and temperament as determinants of early infant crying/fussing behaviour. Pediatrics 84(3), 514-521.

Barr R G, McMullan S J, Speiss H, Leduc D G, Yaremko J, Barfield R, Francoeur T E, Hunziker U A (1991) Carrying as colic 'therapy:' a randomized controlled trial. Pediatrics 87(5), 623-630.

Barr R G, Rotman A, Yaremko J, Leduc D, Francoeur T E (1992) The crying of infants with colic: a controlled empirical description. Pediatrics 90(1), 14-21.

Barr R G, Chen S, Hopkins B, Westra T (1996) Crying patterns in pre-term infants. Developmental Medicine and Child Neurology 38(4), 345-355.

Barr R G, Young S N, Wright J H, Gravel R, Alkawaf R (1999) Differential calming responses to sucrose taste in crying infants with and without colic. Pediatrics 103(5), 1024-1025.

Bartlett L, Witoonchart C (2003) The sleep patterns of young twins. Journal of Family Health Care 13(1), 21-23.

Berkowitz C D, Naveh Y, Berant M (1997) 'Infantile colic' as the sole manifestation of gastroesophageal reflux. Journal of Pediatric Gastroenterology and Nutrition 24(2), 231-233.

Blumenthal I (1997) Use of sucrose as a treatment for infantile colic. Archives of Disease in Childhood 77(4), 370.

Botes S (1998) The CPHVA view of health visiting and the new NHS. Community Practitioner 71(6), 220-222.

Bradford R (1997) Children, Families and Chronic Disease: psychological models and methods of care. London: Routledge.

Brazelton T B (1962) Crying in infancy. Pediatrics 29, 579-588.

Canam C (1993) Common adaptive tasks facing parents of children with chronic conditions. Journal of Advanced Nursing 18(1), 46-53.

Canivet C, Hagander B, Jakobsson I, Lanke J (1996) Infantile colic: less common than previously estimated? Acta Paediatrica 85(4), 454-458.

Canivet C, Jakobsson I, Hagander B (2000) Infantile colic. Follow-up at four years of age: still more 'emotional.' Acta Paediatrica 89(1), 13-17.

Carey W B (1968) Maternal anxiety and infantile colic. Clinical Pediatrics 7(10), 590-595.

Carey W B (1984) 'Colic' – primary excessive crying as an infant–environment interaction. Pediatric Clinics of North America 31(5), 993-1005.

Carey W B (1992) Temperament issues in the school-aged child. Pediatric Clinics of North America 39(3), 569-584.

Carver C S, Scheier M, Weintraub J K (1989) Assessing coping strategies: a theoretically based approach. Journal of Personality and Social Psychology 56(2), 267-283.

Castro-Rodríguez J A, Stern D A, Halonen M, Wright A L, Holberg C J, Taussig L M, Martinez F D (2001) Relation between infantile colic and asthma/atopy: a prospective study in an unselected population. Pediatrics 108(4), 878-882.

Cervisi J, Chapman M, Niklas B, Yamaoka C (1991) Office management of the infant with colic. Journal of Pediatric Health Care 5(4), 184-190.

Chalmers K I, Luker K A (1991) The development of the health visitor–client relationship. Scandinavian Journal of Caring Sciences 5(1), 33-41.

Clifford T J, Campbell M K, Speechley K N, Gorodzinsky F (2003) Sequelae of infant colic: evidence of transient infant distress and absence of lasting effects on maternal mental health. Archives of Pediatrics and Adolescent Medicine 156(12), 1183-1188.

Clyne P S, Kulczycki A (1991) Human breast milk contains bovine IgG. Relationship to infant colic? Pediatrics 87(4), 439-444.

Cody A (1999) Health visiting as therapy: a phenomenological perspective. Journal of Advanced Nursing 29(1), 119-127.

Community Practitioners' and Health Visitors' Association (1997) Public health: the role of nurses and health visitors. London: CPHVA.

Community Practitioners' and Health Visitors' Association (1998) Making the difference: evidence of the effectiveness of health visiting. London: CPHVA.

Crowcroft N S, Strachan D P (1997) The social origins of infant colic: questionnaire study covering 76747 infants. British Medical Journal 314(7090), 1325-1328.

Crowe H P, Zeskind P S (1992) Psycho-physiological and perceptual responses to infant cries varying in pitch: comparison of adults with low and high scores on the Child Abuse Potential Inventory. Child Abuse and Neglect 16(1), 19-29.

Dale B (1997) Parenting and chronic illness. In Altschuler J (Ed) Working with Chronic Illness, pp 111-113, Houndsmill: Macmillan.

Danielsson B, Hwang C P (1985) Treatment of infantile colic with surface active substance (Simethicone). Acta Paediatrica 74(3), 446-450.

DeGangi G, Dipietro J A, Greenspan S I, Porges S W (1991) Psychophysiological characteristics of the regulatory disordered infant. Infant Behaviour and Development 14, 37-50.

Department for Education and Employment (1998) Sure Start. London: HMSO.

Don N, McMahon C, Rossiter C (2002) Effectiveness of an individualised programme for managing unsettled infants. Journal of Paediatrics and Child Health 38(6), 563-567.

Downey J, Bidder R T (1990) Perinatal information on infant crying. Child: Care, Health and Development 16(2), 113-121.

Drotar D, Crawford P (1985) Psychological adaptation of siblings of chronically ill children: research and practical implications. Journal of Developmental and Behavioural Pediatrics 6, 355-362.

Elliott M R, Fisher K, Ames E W (1988) The effects of rocking on the state and respiration of normal and excessive criers. Canadian Journal of Psychology 42(2), 163-172.

Estep D C, Kulczycki A (2000) Treatment of infant colic with amino acid-based infant formula: a preliminary study. Acta Paediatrica 89(1), 22-27.

Field P A (1994) A comparison of symptoms used by mothers and nurses to identify an infant with colic. International Journal of Nursing Studies 31(2), 201-215.

Fish M, Stifter C, Belsky J (1991) Conditions of continuity and discontinuity in infant negative emotionality: newborn to five months. Child Development 62(3), 1525-1537.

Forsyth B W C (1989) Colic and the effect of changing formulas: a double-blind, multiple-crossover study. Journal of Pediatrics 115(4), 521-526.

Frodi A (1985) When empathy fails: aversive infant crying and child abuse. In Lester B M, Boukydis S F (Eds) Infant Crying: theoretical and research perspectives, pp 263-278, New York: Plenum.

Fuller B F (1991) Acoustic discrimination of three types of infant cries. Nursing Research 40(3), 156-160.

Gibson C (1995) The process of empowerment in mothers of chronically ill children. Journal of Advanced Nursing 21(6), 1201-1210.

Gillies C (1987) Infant colic: is there anything new? Journal of Pediatric Health Care 1(6), 305-312.

Golton F, St James-Roberts I (1991) Crying rates in infancy. Health Visitor 64(6), 188-190.

Hall M B (1996) Health for All Children (3rd edn). Oxford University Press.

Heine R G, Jaquiery A, Lubitz L, Cameron D J, Catto-Smith A G (1995) Role of gastro-oesophageal reflux in infant irritability. Archives of Disease in Childhood 73(2), 121-125.

Helseth S (2002) Help in times of crying: nurses' approach to parents with colicky infants. Journal of Advanced Nursing 40(3), 267-274.

Hill D J, Menahem S, Hudson I L, Sheffield L J, Shelton M J, Oberklaid F, Hosking C S (1992) Charting infant distress: an aid to defining colic. Journal of Pediatrics 121(5), 755-758.

Home Office (1998) Supporting Families: a consultation document. London: HMSO.

Hubbard F O A, Van IJzendoorn M H (1991) Maternal unresponsiveness and infant crying across the first 9 months: a naturalistic longitudinal study. Infant Behaviour and Development 14, 299-312.

Huhtala V, Lehtonen L, Heinonen R, Korvenranta H (2000) Infant massage compared with crib vibrator in the treatment of colicky infants. Pediatrics 105(6), E84.

Hunzinker U A, Barr R G (1986) Increased carrying reduces infant crying: a randomized control trial. Pediatrics 77(5), 641-648.

Hyams J S, Geertsma M A, Etienne N L, Treem W R (1989) Colonic hydrogen production in infants with colic. Journal of Pediatrics 115(4), 592-594.

Hymovich D, Hagopian G (1992) Chronic Illness in Children and Adults: a psychosocial approach. London: W B Saunders.

Iacono G, Carroccio A, Montalto G, Cavataio F, Bragion E, Lorello D, Balsamo V, Notarbartolo A (1991) Severe infantile colic and food intolerance: a long-term prospective study. Journal of Pediatric Gastroenterology and Nutrition 12(3), 332-335.

Illingworth C, Timmins J (1990) Gripe water: what is it? Why is it given? Health Visitor 63(11), 378.

Illingworth R S (1954) Three month colic. Archives of Disease in Childhood 29, 165-174.

Illingworth R S (1959) Evening colic in infants: a double-blind trial of dicyclomine hydrochloride. The Lancet 19, 1119-1120.

Illingworth R S (1985) Infantile colic revisited. Archives of Disease in Childhood 60, 981-985.

Jacobson D, Melvin N (1995) A comparison of temperament and maternal bother in infants with and without colic. Journal of Pediatric Nursing 10(3), 181-188.

Jakobsson I, Lindberg T (1983) Cow's milk proteins cause infantile colic in breast-fed infants: a double-blind crossover study. Pediatrics 71(2), 268-271.

Jakobsson I, Lothe L, Ley D, Borschel M W (2000) Effectiveness of casein hydrolysate feedings in infants with colic. Acta Paediatrica 89(1), 18-21.

Jayachandra C (1988) Child Management: five universal basic principles. Penzance: United Writers.

Kalliomäki M, Laippala P, Korvenranta H, Kero P, Isolauri E (2001) Extent of fussing and colic type crying preceding atopic disease. Archives of Disease in Childhood 84(4), 349-350.

Kanabar D, Randhawa M, Clayton P (2001) Improvement in symptoms in infant colic following reduction of lactose load with lactase. Journal of Human Nutrition and Dietetics 14(5), 359-363.

Kearney P J, Malone A J, Hayes T, Cole M, Hyland M (1998) A trial of lactase in the management of infant colic. Journal of Human Nutrition and Dietetics 11(4), 281-285.

Keefe M, Kotzer A M, Froese-Fretz A, Curtin M (1996) A longitudinal comparison of irritable and non-irritable infants. Nursing Research 45(1), 4-9.

Kerr S M, Jowett S A, Smith L N (1996) Preventing sleep problems in infants: a randomized controlled trial. Journal of Advanced Nursing 24(5), 938-942.

Kirjavainen J, Jahnukainen T, Huhtala V, Lehtonen L, Kirjavainen T, Korvenranta H, Mikola H, Kero P (2001) The balance of the autonomic nervous system is normal in colicky infants. Acta Paediatrica 90(3), 250-254.

Lazarus R S, Folkman S (1984) Stress, Appraisal and Coping. New York: Springer.

Lee K (1994) The crying pattern of Korean infants and related factors. Developmental Medicine and Child Neurology 36(7), 601-607.

Lehtonen L A, Korvenranta H (1995) Infantile colic: seasonal incidence and crying profiles. Archives of Pediatrics and Adolescent Medicine 149(5), 533-536.

Lehtonen L A, Korvenranta H, Eerola E (1994a) Intestinal microflora in colicky and non-colicky infants: bacterial cultures and gas-liquid chromatography. Journal of Pediatric Gastroenterology and Nutrition 19(3), 310-314.

Lehtonen L A, Svedstrom E, Korvenranta H (1994b) Gallbladder hypocontractility in infantile colic. Acta Paediatrica 83(11), 1174-1177.

Lester B M, Boukydis C F, Garcia-Coll C T, Hole W T (1990) Colic for developmentalists. Infant Behaviour and Development 15, 15-26.

Lester B M, Boukydis C F, Garcia-Coll C T, Hole W T (1992) Infantile colic: acoustic cry characteristics, maternal perception of cry, and temperament. Infant Mental Health Journal 11, 321-333.

Ley P (1988) Communicating with Parents: improving communication, satisfaction and compliance. London: Chapman.

Lothe L, Lindberg T, Jakobsson I (1982) Cow's milk formula as a cause of infantile colic: a double-blind study. Pediatrics 70(1), 7-10.

Lothe L, Lindberg T, Jakobsson I (1990) Macromolecular absorption in infants with infantile colic. Acta Paediatrica Scandinavica 79(4), 417-421.

Lucassen P L, Assendelft W J, Gubbels J W, Van Eijk J T, Van Geldrop W J, Knuistingh Neven A (1998) Effectiveness of treatments for infantile colic: systematic review. British Medical Journal 316(7144), 1563-1569.

Mangelsdorf S, Gunnar M, Kestenbaum R, Lang S, Andreas D (1990) Infant proneness to distress temperament, maternal personality, and mother infant attachment: associations and goodness of fit. Child Development 61(3), 820-831.

Markestad T (1997) Use of sucrose as a treatment for infantile colic. Archives of Disease in Childhood 76(4), 356-357.

McGlaughlin A, Grayson A (2001) Crying in the first year of infancy: patterns and prevalence. Journal of Reproductive and Infant Psychology 19(1), 47-59.

McKenzie S (1991) Troublesome crying in infants: effect of advice to reduce stimulation. Archives of Disease in Childhood 66(12), 1416-1420.

Medoff-Cooper B (1995) Infant temperament: implications for parenting from birth through one year. Journal of Pediatric Nursing 10(3), 141-145.

Metcalfe T J, Irons T G, Sher L D, Young P C (1994) Simethicone in the treatment of infant colic: a randomized, placebo-controlled, multicenter trial. Pediatrics 94(1), 29-34.

Michelsson K, Rinne A, Paajanen S (1990) Crying, feeding and sleeping patterns in 1 to 12-month-old infants. Child: Care, Health and Development 16(2), 99-111.

Miller A R, Barr R G (1991a) Infantile colic: is it a gut issue? Pediatric Clinics of North America 38(6), 1407-1423.

Miller A R, Barr R G (1991b) Maternal emotional state and infant behaviour: are they related? American Journal of Disease in Childhood 145, 4-21.

Miller J J, Mcveagh P, Fleet G H, Petocz P, Brand J C (1990) Breath hydrogen excretion in infants with colic. Archives of Disease in Childhood 64, 725-729.

Moore D J, Robb T A, Davidson G P (1988) Breath hydrogen response to milk containing lactose in colicky and non-colicky infants. Journal of Pediatrics 113(6), 979-990.

Myers J H, Moro-Sutherland D, Shook J E (1997) Anticholinergic poisoning in colicky infants treated with hyoscyamine sulfate. American Journal of Emergency Medicine 15(5), 532-535.

National Health Service Executive (1999) Review of the Nurses, Midwives and Health Visitors Act: Government response to the recommendations. (HSC 1999/030) London: HMSO.

Neu M, Robinson J (2003) Infants with colic: their childhood characteristics. Journal of Pediatric Nursing 18(1), 12-20.

Oggero R, Garbo G, Savino F, Mostert M (1994) Dietary modification versus dicyclomine hydrochloride in the treatment of severe infantile colics. Acta Paediatrica 83(2), 222-225.

Paradise J (1966) Maternal and other factors in the etiology of infantile colic. Journal of the American Medical Association 197, 123-129.

Parkin P C, Schwartz C J, Manuel B A (1993) Randomized controlled trial of three interventions in the management of persistent crying of infancy. Pediatrics 92(2), 197-201.

Pinyerd B J (1992) Infant colic and maternal health: nursing research and practice concerns. Issues in Comprehensive Pediatric Nursing 15(3), 155-167.

Pritchard P (1986) An infant crying clinic. Health Visitor 59(12), 375-377.

Raiha H, Lehtonen L, Huhtala V, Saleva K, Korvenranta H (2002) Excessively crying infant in the family: mother-infant, father-infant and mother-father interaction. Child: Care, Health and Development 28(5), 419-429.

Reijneveld S A, Brugman E, Hirasing R A (2001) Excessive infant crying: the impact of varying definitions. Pediatrics 108(4), 893-897.

Reust C, Blake R (2000) Diagnostic workup before diagnosing colic. Archives of Family Medicine 9(3), 282-283.

Ruiz-Contreras J, Urquia L, Bastero R (1999) Persistent crying as predominant manifestation of sepsis in infants and newborns. Pediatric Emergency Care 15(2), 113-115.

St James-Roberts I (1989) Persistent crying in infancy. Journal of Child Psychology and Psychiatry 30(2), 189-195.

St James-Roberts I (1991) Persistent infant crying. Archives of Disease in Childhood 66(5), 653-655.

St James-Roberts I (1993a) Infant crying: normal development and persistent crying. In St James-Roberts I, Harris G, Messer D (Eds) Infant crying, feeding and sleeping: development problems and treatments, pp 7-25, Hertfordshire: Harvester Wheatsheaf.

St James-Roberts I (1993b) Explanations of persistent infant crying. In St James-Roberts I, Harris G, Messer D (Eds) Infant crying, feeding and sleeping: development problems and treatments, pp 26-46, Hertfordshire: Harvester Wheatsheaf.

St James-Roberts I, Halil T (1991) Infant crying patterns in the first year: normal community and clinical findings. Journal of Child Psychology and Psychiatry 32(6), 951-968.

St James-Roberts I, Hurry J, Bowyer J (1993) Objective confirmation of crying durations in infants referred for excessive crying. Archives of Disease in Childhood 68(1), 82-84.

St James-Roberts I, Bowyer J, Varghese S, Sawdon J (1994) Infant crying patterns in Manali and London. Child: Care, Health and Development 20(5), 323-337.

St James-Roberts I, Hurry J, Bowyer J, Barr R G (1995) Supplementary carrying compared with advice to increase responsive parenting as interventions to prevent persistent infant crying. Pediatrics 95(3), 381-388.

St James-Roberts I, Conroy S, Wilsher K (1996) Bases for maternal perceptions of infant crying and colic behaviour. Archives of Disease in Childhood 75(5), 375-384.

St James-Roberts I, Sleep J, Morris S, Owen C, Gillham P (2001) Use of a behavioural programme in the first 3 months to prevent infant crying and sleeping problems. Journal of Paediatrics and Child Health 37(3), 289-297.

Sabbeth B, Leventhal J (1984) Marital adjustment to chronic illness: a critique of the literature. Pediatrics 73(6), 762-768.

Søndergaard C, Skajaa E, Henriksen T B (2001) Fetal growth and infantile colic. Archives of Disease in Childhood: Fetal and Neonatal Edition 83(1), F44-F47.

Stahlberg M R, Savilhati E (1986) Infantile colic and feeding. Archives of Disease in Childhood 61, 1232-1233.

Stevens M S (1994) Parents coping with infants requiring home cardiorespiratory monitoring. Journal of Pediatric Nursing 9(1), 2-12.

Taubman B (1984) Clinical trial of the treatment of colic by modification of the parent–infant interaction. Pediatrics 74(6), 998-1003.

Taubman B (1988) Parental counselling compared with elimination of cow's milk or soy milk protein for the treatment of infant colic syndrome: a randomised trial. Pediatrics 81(6), 756-781.

Thomas A, Chess S (1968) The New York longitudinal study: from infancy to early adult life. In Plomin R, Dunn J (Eds) The Study of Temperament: changes, continuities and challenges. Hillsdale, New Jersey: Lawrence Erlbaum.

Thomas A, Chess S (1977) Temperament and Development. New York: Brunner-Mazel.

Thomas A, Chess S, Korn S J (1982) The reality of difficult temperament. Merril-Palmer Quarterly 28(1), 1-20.

Treem W R, Hyams J S, Blankschen E, Etienne N, Paule C L, Borschel M W (1991) Evaluation of a fiber-enriched formula on infant colic. Journal of Pediatrics 119(5), 695-701.

Tyson P D, Sobschak K B (1994) Perceptual responses to infant crying after EEG biofeedback assisted stress management training: implications for physical child abuse. Child Abuse and Neglect 18(11), 933-943.

Van Der Wal M F, Van Den Boom D C, Pauw-Plomp H, De Jonge G A (1998) Mothers' reports of infant crying and soothing in a multicultural population. Archives of Disease in Childhood 79(4), 312-317.

Van IJzendoorn M H, Hubbard F O (2000) Are infant crying and maternal responsiveness during the first year related to infant–mother attachment at 15 months? Attachment and Human Development 2(3), 371-391.

Weissbluth M, Christoffel K K, Davis A T (1984) Treatment of infantile colic with dicyclomine hydrochloride. Journal of Pediatrics 104(6), 951-955.

Weizman Z, Alkrinawi S, Goldfarb D, Bitran C (1993) Efficacy of herbal tea preparation in infantile colic. Journal of Pediatrics 122(4), 650-652.

Wessel M A, Cobb J C, Jackson E B, Harris G S, Detwiler A C (1954) Paroxysmal fussing in infancy: sometimes called 'colic.' Pediatrics 14(5), 421-434.

Whyte D (1997) Family nursing: a systematic approach. In Whyte D (Ed) Explorations in Family Nursing, pp 1-26, London: Routledge.

Wikander B (1995) Nurses' advice to parents with a crying infant. Scandinavian Journal of Caring Sciences 9(2), 87-93

Williams J, Watkin-Jones R (1984) Dicyclomine: worrying symptoms associated with its use in some small babies. British Medical Journal 288, 901.

Wolke D (1993) The treatment of problem crying behaviour. In St James-Roberts I, Harris G, Messer D (Eds) Infant Crying, Feeding and Sleeping: development problems and treatments, pp 47-79, Hertfordshire: Harvester Wheatsheaf.

Wolke D, Gray P, Meyer R (1994) Excessive infant crying: a controlled study of mothers helping mothers. Pediatrics 94(3), 322-332.

Wurmser H, Laubereau B, Hermann M, Paousek M, von Kries R (2001) Excessive infant crying: often not confined to the first 3 months of age. Early Human Development 64(1), 1-6.

Website addresses for cranial osteopathy

The General Osteopathic Council
http://www.osteopathy.org.uk

Osteopathic Centre for Children
http://www.occ.uk.com

The Osteopathic Home Page
http://www.osteohome.com

Website address for Cry-sis

http://www.cry-sis.com

Index